Sueli de Souza Costa

Photodynamic Therapy in Lower Third Molar Alveoli

Sueli de Souza Costa

Photodynamic Therapy in Lower Third Molar Alveoli

Laser in Dentistry

ScienciaScripts

Imprint
Any brand names and product names mentioned in this book are subject to trademark, brand or patent protection and are trademarks or registered trademarks of their respective holders. The use of brand names, product names, common names, trade names, product descriptions etc. even without a particular marking in this work is in no way to be construed to mean that such names may be regarded as unrestricted in respect of trademark and brand protection legislation and could thus be used by anyone.

Cover image: www.ingimage.com

This book is a translation from the original published under ISBN 978-613-9-63758-4.

Publisher:
Sciencia Scripts
is a trademark of
Dodo Books Indian Ocean Ltd. and OmniScriptum S.R.L publishing group

120 High Road, East Finchley, London, N2 9ED, United Kingdom
Str. Armeneasca 28/1, office 1, Chisinau MD-2012, Republic of Moldova, Europe
Printed at: see last page
ISBN: 978-620-7-68851-7

"IF, IN PRINCIPLE, THE IDEA IS NOT ABSURD, THEN THERE IS NO HOPE FOR IT."

ALBERT EINSTEIN

SUMMARY

Photodynamic therapy (PDT) is widely used in medicine to treat tumours, pre-malignant lesions, macular degeneration and psoriasis, and in dentistry it is applied to periodontal pockets, herpes simplex and other microbial lesions. This therapy consists of combining a low-intensity light source with a dye. Bacteria, fungi, yeasts and viruses can also be eliminated by visible light after treatment with an appropriate photosensitiser. Although there have been great advances in the medical field with PDT, there are no known studies of its effect on exodontia. OBJECTIVES: In this study, the effect of PDT on lower third molar alveoli immediately after extraction (experimental side) was analysed "in vivo", compared to extraction without the use of PDT (control). MATERIAL AND METHOD: The dye used was 0.1% methylene blue (AM). Material was collected from the dental alveolus at two times: immediately after exodontia and immediately after the application of photodynamic therapy on the experimental side; and also at two times after exodontia on the control side, with the application of placebo at the second moment. The material collection procedure was repeated after 24 hours. The samples were subjected to culture analysis in the laboratory, and then a comparison was made between exodontia without PDT and exodontia with PDT, associated with a red low intensity laser (LLL), Twin Flex (MM Optics) made of AlGaInP (Indium-Gallium-Aluminium Phosphide), with a wavelength of 660 nm, a power of 40 mW and an energy density of 60 J/cm^2 for 60 seconds. Initially, all the variables were analysed descriptively. For quantitative variables, this analysis was carried out by looking at the minimum and maximum values and calculating means, standard deviations and quartiles (25th percentile, median and 75th percentile). Absolute and relative frequencies were calculated for the qualitative variables. The study involved 13 patients. The significance level used in the statistical tests was 5.0% (0.05). RESULTS: The experimental side showed a drastic reduction in the amount of microorganism growth in both blood and secretion cultures within 24 hours. The experimental side also showed a statistically significant reduction in pain from the first day onwards, greater than the control side. As for oedema, there were differences between the treated and control sides, with a better scar appearance after seven days. The main microorganism isolated in the samples was *Klebsiella* sp, which is responsible for a high mortality rate in immunocompromised individuals. CONCLUSION: For the population studied, PDT proved to be effective and useful in reducing the growth of bacterial colonies in the dental alveolus, reducing pain, oedema and trismus in the post-operative period of lower third molar extraction and facilitating healing, compared to the use of laser alone.

Keywords: Photodynamic Therapy, Methylene Blue, Lasers, Exodontia, *Klebsiella* sp.

SUMMARY

CHAPTER 1

INTRODUCTION: PHOTODYNAMIC THERAPY

Photodynamic Therapy (PDT) is based on the topical or systemic administration of a non-toxic, light-sensitive dye, followed by low-dose irradiation with visible light of an appropriate wavelength. In the presence of oxygen found in cells, the activated photosensitiser (PS) produces reactive species that can react with molecules in its vicinity by two methods: by electron or hydrogen transfer, leading to the production of free radicals (type I reaction) or by energy transfer to oxygen (type II reaction), leading to the production of singlet oxygen, which causes the elimination of the enemy cell (MA; JIANG, 2001; BOYLE, DOLPHIN, 1996), the average lifetime of singlet oxygen in biological systems being less than 40 nanoseconds (ns) (MIAN; BERG, 1991).

When used in conjunction with visible light treatment to eliminate pathogenic microorganisms such as bacteria, yeasts, fungi and viruses, PDT would come to be called Antimicrobial Photodynamic Therapy (MANYAK, 1990; WAINWRIGHT, 1998), in a process known as Photodynamic Inactivation.

Although the main application of PDT is in the treatment of tumours, in the medical field the technique has been used in pre-malignant lesions, age-related macular degeneration and psoriasis, and in dentistry in periodontal pockets, herpes simplex and other lesions of microbial origin.

PDT has made advances in the medical and dental fields. This study verifies "in vivo" the effect of photodynamic therapy immediately after exodontia, using 0.1% methylene blue dye.

This project investigates the presence of bacteria in the dental sockets of lower third molars in the face of the biological activity of photosensitisers belonging to the phenothiazine dye family (methylene blue) when the sockets are sensitised by the dye immediately after extraction and subjected to the action of a low-intensity laser (LLLT).

Laser, on the other hand, is an English acronym for "Light Amplification *by*

Stimulated Emission of Radiation". It is a non-ionising electromagnetic radiation. The function of the laser device changes according to the type of chemical element it uses, being classified as Low Intensity Laser (LLLT) or therapeutic and High Intensity Laser or surgical.

Studies on LLLT on human tissues have been carried out since the 60s, with prospects for its use beginning in the 80s.

Various studies, both in vitro and in vivo, have demonstrated the therapeutic use of LLLT on different types of tissue, ranging from analgesic to anti-inflammatory and trophic-regenerative effects. As a biomodulatory agent, including stimulating soft tissue healing and reducing painful post-surgical symptoms, there are several studies and papers confirming this ability. This is the first study using the administration of LLLTs associated with a photosensitising agent in exodontia.

CHAPTER 2

LITERATURE REVIEW

2.1   The laser

The word "Laser" is an acronym from the English language, *Light Amplification by Stimulated Emission of* Radiation.

The first laser in history was built in 1960 by Theodore Maiman in California, USA (MAIMAN, 1960). It was a ruby laser, operating at 694.3 nanometres (nm). The following year, the first laser laboratory for medical applications was founded at the University of Cincinnati by Leon Goldman (GOLDMAN, 1981), where the first experiments on animals were carried out.

In 1961, Javan et al. developed the Helium-Neon (He-Ne) laser (GENOVESE, 2007). Also in 1961, Patel et al. presented the carbon dioxide laser, emitting radiation in the infrared range, and the following year, the first semiconductor laser (GENOVESE, 2007).

The first clinical applications with low-power lasers were reported in 1966 by Endre Mester, from Hungary, who presented clinical case reports on "Laser Biostimulation" of chronic lower limb ulcers using ruby and argon lasers (MESTER, 1966). He produced a large volume of scientific, clinical and experimental work, with the He-Ne laser as the central theme.

In 1973, Heinrich Plogg, from Fort Coulombe, Canada, along the same lines as Mester, presented a paper entitled "The use of lasers in acupuncture without needles" to minimise pain (BAXTER, 1994). At the end of the 1970s, semiconductor laser diodes began to be developed, giving rise to the first diode operating in the near-infrared region (904nm wavelength), made of gallium arsenide (As-Ga). As well as being smaller than He-Ne, it has greater penetration into biological tissue and can operate in continuous or pulsed mode, whereas He-Ne only operates in continuous mode.

In 1981, there was the first report of the clinical application of an As-Ga-Al (Aluminium Gallium Arsenide) laser diode, published by Calderhead (1981), from Japan, which compared the pain attenuation promoted by a laser diode and the

Nd:YAG laser (Neodynium-Ltri-Aluminium-Garnet), operating at a wavelength of 1064 nm.

Low-intensity lasers have analgesic, anti-inflammatory and biomodulatory effects and are widely used in dentistry for canker sores, fever blisters, angular cheilitis, trismus, paresthesia, dentin hypersensitivity, post-surgery and post-endodontic interventions, causing desirable effects such as increases in local microcirculation and the speed of healing (BRUGNERA JR, PINHEIRO, 1988; DONATO, BORAKS, 1993; GENOVESE, 2007).

2.2 The third molar

According to Peterson (2005), lower third molars are the teeth most commonly involved in infection, especially when they are retained or impacted.

Marzola et al. (1990) stated that the most frequent reason for the retention of mandibular third molars was related to mechanical obstacles (71.7%), in which the poor positioning of neighbouring teeth accounted for the largest percentage (31.3%), followed by the lack of space in the dental arch for irruption (24.5%) and the presence of pathological elements preventing irruption (12.9%). They also noted anterior dental crowding in 47.5% of cases, as well as the association of the third molar with irruption accidents, the majority (52.5%) in the form of damage to the integrity of contiguous teeth, such as root resorption.

Nogueira et al. (1997) point out the most common problems caused by impacted teeth and their clinical solutions. They demonstrate that dental inclusions can cause various health problems, but state that an impacted tooth does not always require removal. And they warn that the earlier the diagnosis and treatment, the less damage caused.

According to Moro et al. (2001), the indications for extraction are infection, cyst formation, pre-irradiation and persistent pain due to unknown causes, the most common being pericoronaritis.

Vasconcellos et al. (2002) explain that retained teeth are those that have not erupted at the correct time, for mechanical or pathological reasons. When evaluating the third molar in its long axis, comparing it with the same axis of the adjacent second molar, out of a total of 1358 third molars, 568 were retained or semi-retained.

Girardi et al. (2004) state that a fully or partially erupted tooth shows the permanence of the reduced epithelium of the enamel organ around the crown, which can lead to various pathologies, with lower third molars being the teeth most affected by eruption problems.

Martorelli et al. (2004) report that complex odontomas behave similarly to impacted teeth and can act as a barrier to their eruption or present inflammatory/infectious processes similar to pericoronaritis.

2.2.1 Post-operative complications

Complications in third molar surgery, according to Larsen (1992) and De Boer et al. (1995), are directly linked to a complicated and prolonged transoperative period. Holland and Hindle (1984) and De Boer (1995) consider surgical technique and operator experience as possible causes, while Larsen (1992) and Chiaspaco (1993) point to the influence of age and gender.

Moro et al. (2001) warn that the post-operative period can be affected by the duration of the procedures, the position of the tooth and the presence of infection.

Calderoni et al. (2003) assessed the incidence of suppurative alveolitis in patients undergoing surgery for 393 mandibular third molars, of which 191 had an open wound and 202 had a closed wound. Eight patients developed suppurative alveolitis, 4 with poor hygiene and 4 with regular hygiene. Alveolitis is a post-exodontic complication characterised by the alveolus being empty or filled with a greyish-yellow layer formed by food debris and necrotic tissue. It is suppurative when there is a purulent secretion rich in bacteria, developing marked pain, a foul odour and swelling.

Gallagher (2003) reports a case of a submasseteric and infratemporal abscess caused by an infected haematoma following the extraction of a third molar, the sequelae of which subsequently resulted in a sensorineural deficit.

Jones et al. (2003) reported two cases of chronic submasseteric abscesses as a result of third molar extraction.

Alveolitis is a common post-operative condition following the extraction of permanent teeth, especially third° molars. The frequency of alveolitis occurs in 1% to 3% of all extractions, rising to 25% to 30% in third molars, and the signs and symptoms can last from 10 to 40 days (CAMNINO, 2003). However, among only cases of alveolitis, they account for 81.25% of extracted lower third molars, according to Vitti et al. (2005).

Pinto et al. (2005) described pericoronaritis as an inflammatory condition of an infectious or non-infectious nature involving the soft tissue covering the crown of a tooth, usually a lower third molar in the process of eruption or semi-inclusion. They report that pericoronaritis can spread, generating more aggressive infectious processes such as septicaemia, osteitis and osteomyelitis, infection of the pleura and mediastinum, infection of the deep fascial spaces and acute necrotising gingivitis. They state that there are significant findings relating pericoronaritis to tonsillitis, and that purulent pharyngeal secretions are more common in tonsillitis in patients who have a partially erupted third molar. They report that because the space between the pericoronal capus and the crown of the partially erupted lower third molar is a reservoir for a variety of microorganisms, extraction of the third molar is indicated, as its removal has been shown to reduce pathogenic microorganisms both at the site and in the oral cavity as a whole. According to the authors, dental pericoronaritis may be related to tonsillitis, and there is even an increase in the frequency of tonsillitis during tooth irruption.

Peterson (2005) is adamant that the most common cause of delayed wound healing is infection, and makes it clear that another clinical condition, alveolar westeritis, can be the result of subclinical infections, reaching 20% of all impacted lower third molar removals.

Cardoso et al. (2008) reported two cases of abscesses three weeks after third molar removal in young patients.

Bortoluzzi et al. (2008), in a retrospective study of 80 patients who underwent third molar removal, found that 13% had teeth removed from the mandibular arch. Of the total, the following complications were found: 2 cases of fibrinolytic alveolitis (2.5%), 2 cases of acute infection (2.5%), 8 cases of significant oedema (10%) and 8 cases of pain lasting more than two days after surgery (10%).

2.2.2 Inflammation and tissue repair

The healing of tooth extraction wounds is no different from the healing of other wounds in the body, except for the peculiar anatomical situation that exists after the tooth has been removed. When tissues are torn, whether by accident or for surgical purposes, a predictable and orderly sequence of biological events takes place (POLLACK, 1979; PEACOCK and WINKLE, 1987).

Healing begins with the formation of a blood clot at the site, and its final organisation is granulation tissue, gradually replaced by coarse fibrillar bone and finally by mature bone. This whole process takes place approximately 5 weeks after tooth extraction and can be visualised radiographically between 6 and 8 weeks.

However, there is always a peculiar inflammatory process, the basic characteristic of which is always the same, i.e. filling space and sealing it with a scar. The first 24 hours after the injury are extremely important in determining how healing will take place. For Manjo and Joris (1996), the presence of bacteria, the degree of blood supply, the nature of the wound (open or closed), the amount of dead tissue to be eliminated, the type of tissue injured and other factors determine how healing will occur. There is better healing when the wound is closed, sutured and not infected, known as an incisional wound, where the healing process progresses directly to the production of a scar; in contrast to the situation in which an excisional wound occurs, where a fragment of tissue is removed.

Cases of infection and protein loss can occur during the wound repair process, according to Stockausen and Felbier (1972).

2.3 Photosensitisers

According to Perussi (2007), the photosensitisers that have been studied for eradicating microorganisms belong to different groups of compounds, such as halogenated xanthenes, such as Rose Bengal (RB); phenothiazines, such as toluidine blue O (ATO) and methylene blue (AM); acridines, and chlorine conjugates (e6) (WAINWRIGHT, 2002).

The synthesis of the phenothiazine dye Methylene Blue was described by Caro in 1876, at the time of the industrial boom, and it was used mainly as a dye for fabrics at that time (PELOI, 2007). It was used as an antimalarial drug by Ehrlich 15 years later.

In terms of drug research, chemically, the phenothiazine ring system is one of the longest-established heterocycles, allowing for a better understanding of the chemical synthesis of phenothiazines, and easy preparation of analogues (Figure 1).

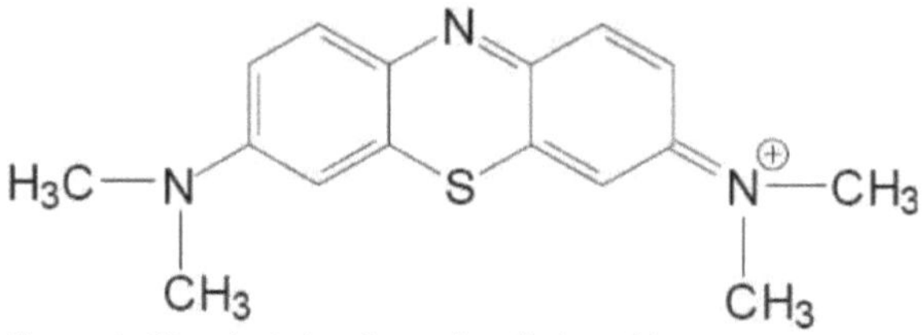

Figure 1: Chemical structure of methylene blue

When applied to cells, it is well established that the AM cation intercalates into the nucleic acid (DNA) structure due to the positive charge and sufficient planar surface area of the photosensitiser in question (WAINWRIGHT, 2002). AM accumulates preferentially in the mitochondria of cells, as these contain a variety of proteins in their membrane, and their selectivity is determined by lipophilicity and charge, which if positive is attracted due to the negative electrochemical environment of the mitochondrial matrix (GABRIELLE et al., 2004).

But this chromophore is easily reduced by biological systems and therefore its antibacterial activity is low. Both in cancer PDT and in recent antimicrobial regimens, commercial phenothiazine dyes have shown the disadvantage of inherent toxicity (in the dark), which causes a decrease in therapeutic efficiency (PERUSSI, 2007). Therefore, rational development studies have been carried out for the synthesis of AM analogues (TARDIVO et al., 2005; FUKUDA et al., 1993).

Despite this, a comparative study of AM cytotoxicity in the dark in normal and tumour cells found that this dye is more cytotoxic in tumour cells (KIRSZBERG et al., 2005; MENEZES et al., 2007). The fact that both MDR (macular degeneration of the retina) cells and strains of bacteria resistant to multiple antibiotics are also sensitive to the dye (DEMIDOVA et al., 2004) suggests that AM can be used as a chemotherapeutic agent.

Methylene blue has been used clinically to treat bladder cancer, inoperable oesophageal tumours, skin virulence, psoriasis and adenocarcinomas (ORTH et al., 1995). It is also used as a photosensitiser in viral blood disinfection, being one of the very few sterilisation methods known to date that can be successful on red blood cell concentrates (BESSELINK et al., 2003), as it is effective in inactivating viruses including HIV/AIDS, hepatitis B and C (FLOYD et al., 2004; WAINWRIGHT, 2000). The dengue virus can also be eradicated by AM and PDT (HUANG et aL, 2004).

The main targets for PDT in mammalian cells are lysosomes, mitochondria and plasma membranes, while in microbial cells damage to the outer membrane plays an important role by preventing DNA damage. It can be used topically in infections in non-perfused tissues, such as burns, and may have less toxicity when compared to other topical antimicrobial treatments (DEMIDOVA et al., 2004).

Phenothiazine dyes exhibit intense absorption at a wavelength of 600-660 nm, a region of the spectrum that is useful in PDT because it is in the "therapeutic window" required for efficient penetration of light into tissues (WAINWRIGHT et al., 1999; STERNBERG et al., 1998; STERNBERG and DOLPHIN, 1996). According to Tardivo et al. (2005), AM in aqueous solution is present in the form of monomers (dilute solutions), dimers and larger aggregates (very concentrated solutions), which can be distinguished by their absorption bands, maxima at 664nm, 600nm and in the region of 550 nm, respectively.

Methylene blue has recently been considered as a drug for PDT (TARDIVO et al., 2005; ITRI, 2002) as it has shown in vivo activity against various types of tumour when used in PDT.

The mechanism of action of AM under a light source occurs in the presence of oxygen found in cells, when the activated photosensitiser (PS) can react with molecules in its vicinity by transferring electrons or hydrogen, leading to the production of free radicals (type I reaction) or by transferring energy to oxygen, leading to the production of singlet oxygen (type II reaction). On the other hand, when AM is activated to the excited singlet state (^{1} AM*), it can, with equal probability, return to the singlet state or go to the triplet state (^{3} AM*). If triplet, AM can react with O2 to form singlet oxygen (O^1_2) and return to its normal state or, in a much slower process, form superoxide. Alternatively[3] AM* can react with substrates generating reactive oxygen species (FLOYD et al., 2004). Both pathways can lead to cell apoptosis and the destruction of diseased tissue (LAMBRECHTS et al., 2005; DEMIDOVA et al., 2005).

For the drug (photosensitiser) to be commercially viable and effective in its therapeutic action, it must meet a set of favourable properties (STEMBERG et al., 1998; SIMPLÍCI et al., 2002):

i) favourable photophysical characteristics;

ii) low toxicity in the dark (low cytotoxicity);

iii) non-prolonged photosensitivity;

iv) simplicity of formulation, reproducibility and high stability of the formulation;

v) favourable pharmacokinetics (rapid elimination from the body);

vi) ease of synthetic handling that allows modifications to be made to optimise the desired properties;

vii) easy to obtain on an industrial scale at low cost and with good reproducibility;

viii) the facility to fully analyse the components of the formula, including the provision of validation scripts, and

ix) high affinity and penetration into diseased tissue to the detriment of healthy tissue (selectivity).

Among the important photophysical properties, these compounds must not undergo photobleaching reactions (photodegradation), as the chromophore would be undergoing chemical modifications in such a way that the light absorption process would be altered and the effectiveness of subsequent photochemical processes would be diminished. Another characteristic is its high hydrophobicity, a property that makes it easier to interact with biological targets, including cell membranes (STERNBERG et al., 1998). This characteristic, however, gives the molecules a high tendency to self-aggregate in aqueous solution and, in the aggregated state, the drug reduces the production of singlet oxygen (due to the rapid deactivation of energy from excited states by the self-suppression phenomenon), which could compromise the efficiency of the treatment (STERNBERG et al., 1998; MACHADO, 2000).

2.3.1 Light sources used in TFD

Various light sources can be used to activate the photosensitiser, such as pulsed light, incoherent lights (slide projectors), xenon lamps, among others, all with specific filters that make it possible to select the wavelength of greatest penetration into the tissues and maximum absorption of the drug (PELOI, 2007). In photodynamic therapy, the radiation used is generally provided by a laser system that is directed to the treatment site via optical fibres.

Laser beams are favoured because they have three characteristics that differentiate them from ordinary light: the light is monochromatic (a single wavelength), coherent (single phase) and unidirectional (collimated beam), and laser systems can also be powerful (GENOVESE, 2007). The radiation density in PDT is given in J/cm^2. A variety of lasers can be used, depending on the characteristics and stage of the lesion.

In this work, a red, Twin Flex (MM Optics Ltda, São Carlos, S.P. Brazil) AlGaInP (Indium-Gallium-Aluminium Phosphide) low-intensity laser (LBI) was used, with a wavelength of 660 nm, a beam area of 0.04 cm^2, at a power of 40 mW, and an energy density of 60 J/cm^2 for 60 seconds.

2.3.2 Photodynamic therapy (PDT) and the laser

Photodynamic therapy is highly effective in reducing cell death in experimental procedures and has been used to induce the elimination of pathogenic microorganisms.

The use of light in therapy has been known for more than three millennia, used in the treatment of vitiligo by the Indians (ACKROYD et al., 2001). However, it was only in 1900 that Oscar Raab, in Munich, observed the death of infusoria, a species of paramecium, when exposed to certain wavelengths of light in the presence of acridine red, describing the concept of cell death induced by the interaction of chemical substances and light. The Frenchman J. Prime (1901) treated a patient's epilepsy by applying eosin orally, which induced dermatitis in the areas exposed to sunlight. Von Tappeiner and A. Jesionek (1903) used topical eosin and white light to treat skin tumours. VonTappeiner and Jodlbauer (1904) demonstrated the need for the presence of oxygen for the reaction to occur, and described this effect in 1907 as photodynamic action.

Since then, various experiments have been carried out to assess the effects of photosensitivity and phototoxicity, pharmacodynamics and pharmacokinetics of photosensitisers, proving the efficacy of PDT.

One of the advantages of PDT compared to the use of traditional antimicrobial agents is that bacterial elimination is achieved in a shorter period of time, and it is not necessary to maintain the photosensitiser in high concentrations in the target area for long periods of time (MALIK et al., 1990).

Wilson and Dobson (1992) and Ferreira (2003) carried out studies showing that many bacteria in the oral cavity, including periodontopathogenic bacteria, are susceptible to toluidine blue as a photosensitising agent in photodynamic therapy. But this is only possible when oxygen is present at the site to be treated, as the toxic radicals that will destroy the bacteria are formed from it in PDT (TOMÉ, 2002). As most bacterial species do not have photosensitive components, it is necessary to use a compound that attracts light and initiates the formation of free radicals (WILSON et al., 1992).

Hass et al. (1997) carried out an "in vitro" study to evaluate the effectiveness of PDT on bacteria on the polished surface of titanium discs contaminated with *Porphyromonas gingivalis, Prevotela intermédia and Actinobacilos actinomycetemcomitans,* and concluded that toluidine blue at a concentration of 100 µg/mL, applied before the use of a 905 nm diode laser, in pulsed mode, at 7.3 mW of power, for 60 seconds, was effective in eliminating them.

Walsh (1997), analysing deep caries cavities in teeth colonised by pathogenic microorganisms from the oral flora, points out that if PDT is used, bacterial elimination occurs with little or no risk of damage to the dental pulp or periodontal ligament and that if only laser treatment or only treatment with dyes is carried out, the effect produced on the bacteria is minimal.

Athiré (2002) showed a reduction in the inflammatory process with the application of an aluminium gallium arsenide laser (λ = 830nm) in the post-operative period in the region of exodontia of included or semi-included lower third molars, but without using the PDT technique. He used 5 patients who underwent surgery on both the right and left sides at different times. In the first stage, surgery was carried out on one of the teeth in the conventional manner without the use of LLLT, and the inflammatory process was checked on days 1° , 3° and 7, *which were* considered control elements. In a second stage, 21 days after the first surgery, the homologous dental element was extracted, following the same technique as before and adding low-intensity laser irradiation with an application of 4 J/cm^2 at 4 points, in the immediate post-operative period, 1° and 3° days, observing and monitoring the inflammatory process, as well as measuring these in the post-operative period, 1° , 3° and 7° days, this side being considered experimental (side with laser application).

Athiré (2002) observed that there was a statistically significant reduction in oedema, pain and colour on the side where the laser was applied, compared to the control side.

Lima (2004) carried out a histological study, checking the repair of delayed cutaneous wounds caused on the backs of rats using heated puch and submitted to treatment with low intensity laser, associated or not with the photosensitising drug Toluidine Blue (ATO). In his study, he found that LLLT associated with ATO promoted a reduction in inflammatory infiltrate, great epithelial differentiation, greater collagen deposition and a reduction in wound healing time. He concluded that LLLT and photodynamic therapy act as coadjuvant biostimulatory agents, balancing out the undesirable effects of the wound healing process.

Ribeiro and Zezel (2004) emphasise that PDT techniques have great potential to be explored, as they are low-cost for the treatment of local diseases and infections and cause minimal alterations to surrounding tissues.

Meisel and Kocher (2005) emphasise that although PDT is still at an experimental stage of development and testing, it can be an adjunct to conventional antimicrobial therapy in periodontics.

Hashimoto (2005) proved bacterial reduction with blue light emitting diodes associated with the photosensitiser rhodamine acid B (in PDT), through an *in vitro* study on *Streptococcus mutans, a* common bacterium in oral flora.

In an *in-vitro* study, Prates (2005) used malachite green (MV) as a photosensitiser in photodynamic therapy to check its bactericidal action on *Actinobacillus actinomycetemcomitans, a* microorganism in the subgingival biofilm on the surface of teeth, concluding that this microorganism is photosensitised and eliminated by the combination of *laser* and MV, and the dye is photodegraded after irradiation.

Muller (2006) analysed the effectiveness of the photosensitisers methylene blue (at a concentration of 5.34 ug/mL) and chloro-aluminium phthalocyanine tetrasulphonate (AIPcS4) (at concentrations of 10 ug/mL, 20 ug/mL, 30 ug/mL AND 40 ug/mL) on gram + bacterial strains *{Staphiilococcus aureus, Enterococcus faecalis, Streptococcus mutans)*, concluding that both were effective in leading to bacterial apoptosis in photodynamic therapy. It also showed that methylene blue also promotes significant reductions in all the bacteria studied, even without laser irradiation.

Zancanella et al. (2005) carried out a comparative study between methylene blue and zinc phthalocyanine in the inactivation of *Streptococus aureus,* concluding that the latter was slightly more effective than the former, and that both represented an alternative procedure to antibiotic therapy. Komerik and Macrobert (2006) emphasise that PDT has the potential to establish itself as an excellent alternative treatment for infections of the oral cavity.

According to Peloi (2007), even with the use of LED light to activate methylene blue, there is a photodegradation effect on strains of certain bacteria. The photodynamic effect was tested on *Staphylococcus aureus, Escherichia coli,*

Candida albicans and Artemia salina, and the strains studied suffered an inhibitory effect on growth and mortality in the presence of methylene blue, which was intensified with the application of LED light.

Schwingel (2007) evaluated the efficacy of antimicrobial photodynamic therapy in the treatment of candidiasis in HIV-positive patients, using methylene blue at a concentration of 450 ug/mL in distilled water and a pre-irradiation time of 1 min, comparing it with conventional medication for candidosis (Fluconazole 100mg a day for 14 days) and with a group irradiated with a low-power laser with a wavelength of 660nm, power of 30mW and energy density of $7.5J/cm^2$, in contact with the mucosa for 10 s per affected point. He concluded that antimicrobial photodynamic therapy was promising, as it eradicated 100% of *Candida sp* colonies and showed no recurrence of the disease up to 30 days after irradiation.

A) Exposure time

Wainwright (1998) warns that when methylene blue and toluidine blue dyes are used, it is important to expose the target tissue to the dye in PDT before exposing it to light radiation.

The pre-sensitisation period of the photosensitiser to the laser beam in antimicrobial PDT ranges from one to ten minutes (RIBEIRO et al, 2005).

Marinho (2006) used a five-minute period of pre-sensitisation of methylene blue to laser application on strains of *Candida sp,* showing satisfactory results.

Soukos et al. (2006), using methylene blue (AM) for five minutes, followed by exposure to laser light, on *Enterococus faecalis* in experimental dental canals, proved bacterial reduction and concluded that PDT can be an adjunct to endodontic treatment.

Similar work and results were also reported by Foschi et al. (2007).

Fontana (2007) used methylene blue for five minutes on samples of bacteria from the subgingival plaque of patients with chronic periodontitis, concluding that MA can be an adjunct to periodontal treatment.

Garcez et al. (2003) present a table listing authors, wavelengths used, types of dyes, concentrations, irradiation time and microorganisms tested. Citing methylene blue, they point to experiments by Wilson et al. in 1993, with a wavelength of 632.8 nm, a concentration of 0.025% and irradiation times of 10 seconds, 20 s, 40 s, 80 s, with the microorganism S. *Sanguis. He* also mentions Ovchinnikov who, in 2001, carried out an experiment with AM at 0.1%, for 120 s, at a wavelength of 632.8nm, with the microorganism *Staphylococcus.* Wilson did the same in 1993 with 0.025% AM for 80 seconds on the microorganism *P.gingivalis.*

Almeida et al. in 2006 cited Chan and Lai who, in 2003, used 0.01% AM at a wavelength of 830 nm, with a density of 21.2 J/cm^2 for 60 seconds, proving to be 99-100% effective against *Porphyromonas gingivalis* and *Prevotella Intermedia.*

Schwingel (2007) carried out an experiment on HIV-positive patients with oral candidosis, using AM at a concentration of 450 ug/mL, with a pre-irradiation time of 1 minute, and a low-power laser of 660 nm, 30 mW, 7.5 J/cm^2 por w seconds per affected point, concluding that it had eradicated 100% of the colonies of fungi of the genus *Candida sp.*

In this study, methylene blue remained in contact with the dental alveolus for five minutes before the laser was applied.

2.4 Oral microbiota

The human oral microbiota is highly complex and diverse, characterised by the presence of around 400 bacterial species, as well as fungi, protozoa, mycoplasmas and viruses (MARCOTTE and LAVOIE, 1998).

Some microorganisms, such as *Actinobacillus ctinomycetemcomitans, Bacteroides forsythus* and *Porphyromonas gingivalis* have ample evidence as to their specificity as etiological agents of periodontitis (ZAMBON, 1996).

The salivary level of *mutans* streptococci has been used as an indicator of caries risk (ROSA, 1994; NEWBRUN et al., 1984; KOHLER et al., 1981). Scannapieco and Mylotte (1996) studied the relationship between periodontal problems and bacteria that cause pneumonia.

Santos and Jorge (1999) found that bacteria from the *Enterobacteriaceae P Pseudomonadaceae* families can act as aggravating factors in some types of periodontal disease, including K. *pneumoniae* and *K.oxyutoca, which* have a high incidence rate in the oral cavity.

Okoje et al. (2006) found a predominance of coliforms (Klebsiella spp (15.8%), E. *Coli (13.7%))* in the microbiota isolated from oral mucosa, compared to the normal flora (6.6%). In caries cavities, they also found a predominance of coliforms: *E.Coli* (20.6%), *Klebsiella sp (12.0%)*, *Proteus* (8.6%); with 10.34% of the flora considered normal.

Pimenta et al. (2006) isolated, counted and identified bacteria present in the saliva of children attending a social programme in Goiânia. They found 63 *mutans* group *Streptococcus (MGS)* (95.5 per cent); 38 S. *aureus* (55.0 per cent) and 21 *Coagulase Negative Staphylococci (*30.0 per cent); 13 non-fermenting gran-negative rods (GNB) (29.9 per cent); 8 *Klebsiella pneumoniae* (18.4 per cent), 7 *Enterobacter aerogenes (*16 per cent), 1 *Shigella sonnei (2.3 Es* and 1 *Escherichia coli (2.3* per cent). Most of the EGM and staphylococci had counts of more than 100,000 cfu/mL, while the BGN ranged from 25 cfu/mL to 575 cfu/mL. They report that the presence of *Staphylococcus sp* and *Klebsiella pneumoniae* in the mouth is extremely important, as they can act as supplementary microbiota and in certain situations cause oral or systemic disease.

Caliceti (1948) found *Streptococcus pyogenes* in the buccopharyngeal cavity, where it ranks first among all germs and in 50% to 55% of cases is haemolytic streptococcus.

Christoffersen and Richtner (1951) studied 268 cases of chronic tonsillitis bacteriologically, with the following results: *Streptococcus* (unidentified) 75%, Streptococcus *pyogenes* 25%, *Streptococcus* (inert) 15%, *Staphylococcus aureus 2tEo, Staphylococcus albus* 23%, *Escherichia coli* 6%.

Mion (1965) studied the bacterial flora in tonsillar and focal pathology and found common bacteria in the mouth, such as *Staphylococcus aureus* (plasmo-coagulase positive) and *Streptococcus pyogenes.*

Since the 1970s and 1980s, some authors have identified bacteria present in dental biofilm that could colonise the oropharyngeal cavity (WIKSTROM; LINDE, 1986; GIBBONS, 1989; JOHANSON et al., 1969).

Fourrier, et al (1998), observed that after five days in the ICU, patients who developed nosocomial pneumonia had their bacterial aetiology associated with the bacterial composition of dental plaque.

Bacteria of oral origin reach the lower respiratory tract by haematogenous diffusion and aspiration (FINEGOLD, 1991; *The committee for The Japanese Respiratory Society guidelines in management of respiratory infections Respirology,* 2004).

Haematogenous diffusion of bacteria is rare, with only two cases documented in the literature (MORRIS; SEWELL, 1994; CHRISTENSEN et al, 1993). On the other hand, aspiration of microorganisms from the upper airways during sleep occurs in 45% of healthy patients and 70% of alcoholics, drug users and epileptics (HUXLEY et al., 1978).

Other authors prefer to explain how microorganisms can contaminate the lower respiratory tract via possible routes:

1) aspiration of the contents of the oropharynx (SINCLAIR; EVANS, 1994);

2) inhalation of infected aerosols (TOEWS, 1986);

3) spread of infection through contiguous areas (MOJON, 2002);

4) haematogenous spread through infectious areas extrapulmonary (e.g. gastrointestinal tract infection) (BUENO-CAVANILLAS et al., 1994; SCANNAPIECO et al., 2003).

Three possible mechanisms for associating oral biofilm with respiratory infections are also pointed out:

1) oral biofilm with poor hygiene (SOCRANSKY et al., 1963; CONTRERAS, SLOTS, 2000) would result in a high concentration of pathogens in the saliva, which could be aspirated into the lungs in large quantities, deteriorating immune defences (MANGANIELLO et al., 1977; SCANNAPIECO et al., 1992);

2) due to specific conditions, the oral biofilm could harbour colonies of lung pathogens and promote their growth (FUXENCH-LOPEZ, RAMIREZ-RONDA,1978; WIKSTROM, LINDE, 1986);

3) the bacteria present in oral biofilm could facilitate colonisation of the

upper airways by pulmonary pathogens (MOJON, 2002; SCANNAPIECO et al, 2003).

Oliveira et al. (2007), investigating the presence of respiratory pathogens in the oral cavity of ICU patients, found that the bacteria most frequently found in the patients' tracheal aspirate were *S. pneumoniae* 23.3% (7), *P. aeruginosa* 20% (6), *S. aureus* 13.3% (4), *Kleibsella pneumoniae* 13.3% (4), *Candida albicans* 6.6% (2), *Streptococcus a-hemolytic* 6.6% (2), *Staphylococcus* sp. 6.6% (2), *Aoinetobaoter oalooaoetious - baumanii oomplex (A. oalooaoetious)* in 1 patient (3.3% of all patients), *Esoheriohia ooli (E.ooli)* 3.3% (1), *Enterobaoter oloaoae (E. oloaoae)* 3.3% (1). In these patients, 70% of these bacteria were found in the dental biofilm, 63.33% in tongue samples, 73.33% in artificial respirator tube samples and in 43.33% in all areas simultaneously.

Santos (2007) assessed the prevalence, sensitivity profile and genetic variety of ESBL (extended spectrum P - lactamase) producing *Klebsiella pneumoniae* samples in a hospital in Goiânia, where
found a high prevalence of ESBL-producing *Klebsiella pneumoniae* samples (25 per cent, 28.5 per cent and 66.7 per cent respectively) and resistance rates to β-lactam antimicrobials were higher among isolates producing extended-spectrum β-lactamases (ESBL).

2.4.1 The genus *Klebsiella*

Microorganisms of the genus *Klebsiella* are found in almost all natural environments (soil, water and plants), having initially been isolated in plants and not associated with infections. However, clinical isolates of *K. planticola have* been described in relation to infections causing sepsis. Isolated strains of *K. planticola* and *K. pneumoniae* have been isolated from rice and other plant species, but the majority of clinical isolates belong to the *K. pneumoniae, K. oxytoca* and *K. granulomatis* species (ROLLINS and JOSEPH, 2000).

K. pneumoniae has been isolated from the mouth of individuals with or without periodontal disease and in the oropharynx of asymptomatic carriers. Colonisation of the oropharynx is a source of pulmonary infections in patients debilitated by alcoholism, diabetes, chronic lung diseases or with a depressed immune system, and is responsible for a high mortality rate. Among the most frequent clinical syndromes are pneumonia, urinary tract and wound infections, bacteraemia, chronic atrophic rhinitis, arthritis, enteritis, meningitis in children and sepsis (MADSON et al., 1994; INGHAM, 2000). Most clinical isolates of *K. pneumoniae* are encapsulated and have great pathogenic potential (SAHLY et al., 2002).

Brazilian studies are limited to a few cities. At Hospital São Paulo, a teaching hospital of the Federal University of São Paulo, Gales (1997) found a prevalence of ESBL-producing *K. pneumoniae of* 39 per cent; while Marra (2002) found that 39 per cent of *K. pneumoniae* strains isolated from the bloodstream were ESBL-producing.

Also in this hospital, Carmo Filho (2003) showed that the prevalence of infections caused by *K. pneumoniae* in the adult ICU was 31 per cent, of which 69 per cent were ESBL producers, and in the neonatal ICU, the prevalence was 53.8 per cent, of which 46.2 per cent were ESBL producers.

According to Oliveira et al. (2007), the presence of respiratory pathogens in the oral biofilm of ICU patients can serve as a reservoir for micro-organisms associated with nosocomial pneumonia. They also report that among all hospital-acquired infections, nosocomial pneumonia is responsible for 10% to 15% of this total; and 20% to 50% of all patients affected by infections die.

CHAPTER 3

PROPOSAL:

The aim of this study was to comparatively analyse the effects of photodynamic therapy on the alveoli of homologous mandibular third molars.

CHAPTER 4

MATERIAL AND METHOD

4.1 Material

The following materials were used: Sterile 0.1% methylene blue; 9 ml Haemocult I (Paediatric) culture medium; Swab with culture medium; Sterile gloves; Masks; Caps; Sterile gauze; Paper towels; Liquid soap; Disposable surgical field; Disposable short and long gum needles; Sterile, disposable 3 cc hypodermic syringes and needles.Injectable anaesthetic, Lidocaine 2% with phenylephrine; Scalpel blades n° 12 and 15; 4-0 needle silk thread; Povedine; PVPI; Chlorhexidine 0.12%; Disposable dental surgical sucker; Sterile saline solution; Mouth mirror with handle; Carpule syringe; Steel tray; Clinical forceps; Gouge forceps; Curved and straight haemostatic forceps; Muller bone file; No. 3 scalpel handle; Mayo-Hegar needle holder; Faraboeuf and Minessota retractors; Surgical scissors; Exodontic forceps; Seldin and apical levers; No. 7 spatula or Mead periosteum detacher; Curettes; Zecrya drill; Twin Flex (MM Optics) AlGaInP (Indium-Gallium-Aluminium Phosphide) low-intensity red laser; dental chair; High-rotation motor.

4.2 Method

4.2.1 Patient selection

After approval by the Human Research Ethics Committee of the Cruzeiro do Sul University, 13 volunteer patients were selected, 11 of whom were female, all healthy, aged between 16 and 29 years, with lower third molar teeth that were homologous in terms of position and degree of development, indicated for extraction, on both the right and left sides of the mouth, so that there could be comparisons between the experimental and control sides.

The Informed Consent Form was signed by the patients and/or legal guardians, after clarifications had been made regarding the benefits and risks of using photodynamic therapy and low-intensity lasers in the proposed procedures, in accordance with current legislation.

After the clinical examination of the patients, nothing was diagnosed that would contraindicate the proposed tooth extraction surgery in the volunteers who agreed to take part.

The patients selected had third molars with indications for extraction (Figure 2), following the classic indications, mainly in terms of suitability for orthodontic treatment, a history of pericoronaritis and TMD.

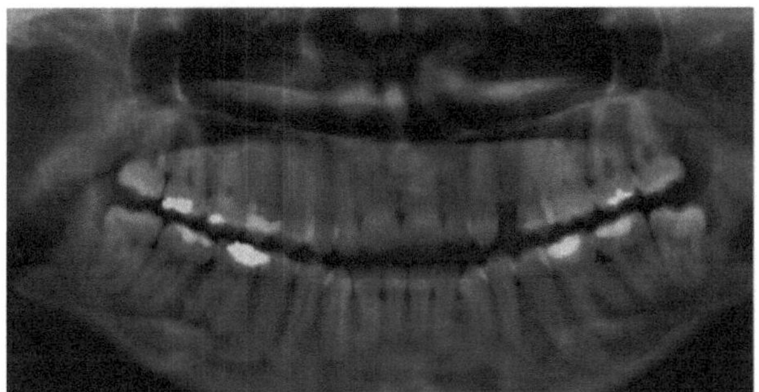

Figure 2: Panoramic radiograph showing homologous lower molars

4.2.2 Surgical technique and experiment

The surgical technique used is traditional (GRAZIANI, 1976; MARZOLA, 1994; GREGORI, 2004), with an estimated duration of one hour for each extracted element, using instruments sterilised in an autoclave and patients degermed with 0.12% chlorhexidine.

Both third molars of each patient's mandibular arch were extracted in the same session (Figures 3 and 4).

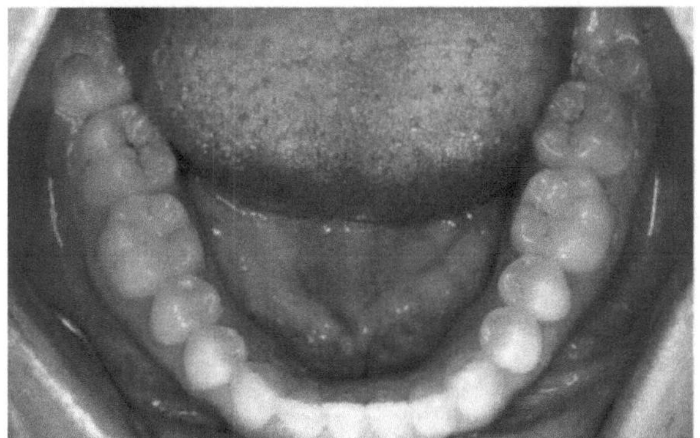

Figure 3: Oral cavity before surgery: teeth 48 and 38

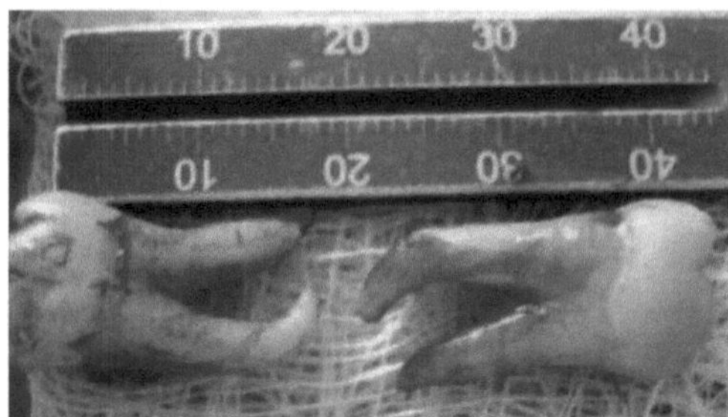
Figure 4: teeth 48 and 38

Two to three tubes of anaesthetic were used on each side, blocking the inferior alveolar nerve, complementing the lingual and buccal branches, as well as using intraseptal and intraligamentary anaesthesia.

Winter's incision was used on both sides of the lower arch of the same patient, when indicated.

Odontosection was carried out, when indicated, on both sides of the mandibular arch of the same patient, considering the homologous situation of both mandibular third molars. Odontosection was carried out with a Zecrya drill in the vestibulo-lingual direction of the dental crown in order to separate the tooth into two parts and facilitate its complete removal.

The actual extraction was carried out after the tooth was dislocated using lifts.

The surgical site was treated in two ways:

1- For the experimental side, tooth 48 was chosen, as it was the first side to undergo surgery in all the selected patients. On the experimental side, 1 cc of blood was immediately collected from the dental alveolus using a hypodermic needle syringe and immediately inoculated into a blood culture medium to be sent to the appropriate laboratory (Blood Culture 1). Then

0.1% methylene, filling the entire alveolar cavity. The patient waited five minutes and then the low-intensity red laser light (LLL), emitted by the Twin Flex (MM Optics Ltda, São Carlos, S. P. Brazil) AlGaInP (Indium-Gallium-Aluminium Phosphide) device, with a wavelength of 660 nm, a power of 40 mW, a beam area of 0.04 cm^2 and an energy density of 60 J/cm^2 was applied to the alveolus for 60 seconds (Figure 5). The area was irrigated abundantly with saline solution in order to remove the methylene blue used and a new 1 cc blood sample was taken from the same site (Blood Culture 3) for examination in the laboratory. The wound was irrigated again with saline solution and sutured with needlepoint silk thread.

2- On the control side (tooth 38), 1 cc of blood was collected immediately after extraction from the socket using a hypodermic needle syringe, for examination (Haemoculture 2) in an appropriate laboratory, followed by the application of placebo for five minutes. LLLT was applied to the socket under the same conditions as the experimental side, followed by irrigation with saline and the collection of a further 1 cc of blood. Then suturing was carried out with needle silk thread.

The patients were not medicated, given the analgesic, anti-inflammatory and biomodulatory effects of the laser. However, they were instructed to apply ice internally and externally to the surgical site for 15 minutes, four times in the first 24 hours, on both sides of the mouth, and to rest. They were also instructed to return to the consulting room within 24 hours.

All the 1 cc blood samples collected using a hypodermic syringe were immediately inoculated into vials containing 9 ml of paediatric Hemocult I culture medium (Figure 6), capable of recovering demanding and non-requiring microorganisms, according to the manufacturer (Laborclin).

According to the manufacturer, the culture medium is intended to be used as a culture medium for isolating microorganisms from blood samples (Laborclin). The culture medium is made up of 9 ml of TSB (Tryptic Soy Broth) medium to inoculate 1 ml of blood, with the addition of SPS (Sodium Polyanethol Sulphonate), which acts as an anticoagulant and inhibits the activity of complement and lysozyme, thus interfering with the phagocytosis process; CO_2 and a vacuum that ensures anaerobic conditions until the moment of inoculation of the collected material.

All the samples were immediately sent to a specialised laboratory for blood culture.

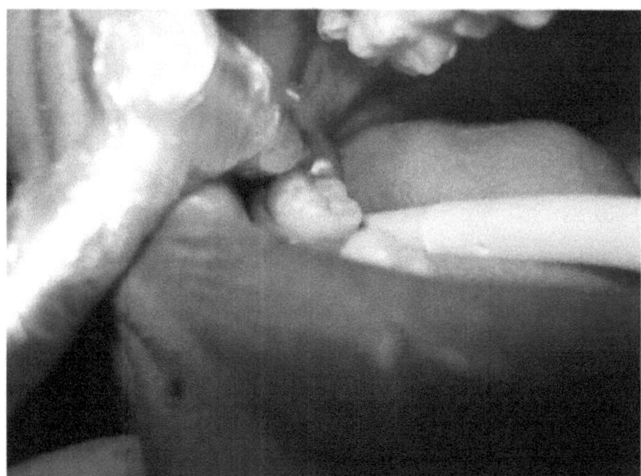
Figure 5: Laser application on methylene blue

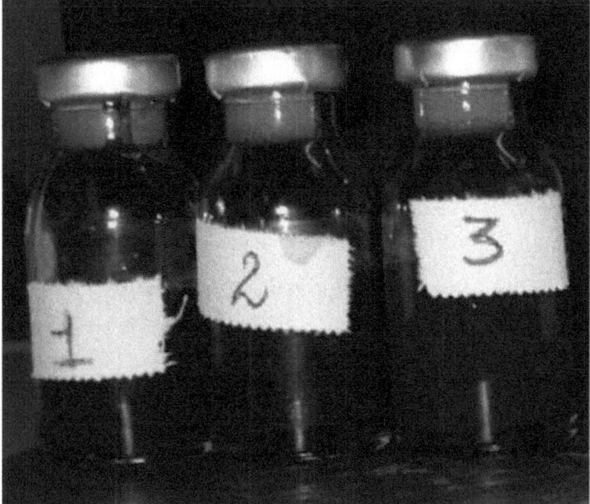
Figure 6: Samples 1, 2, 3, for blood culture (at the time of collection)

The day after the extractions, clinical follow-up was carried out, when the degree of pain reported by the patient on both surgical sides was checked using the Virtual Analogue Scale (VAS), from 0 to 10 points (Figure 7).

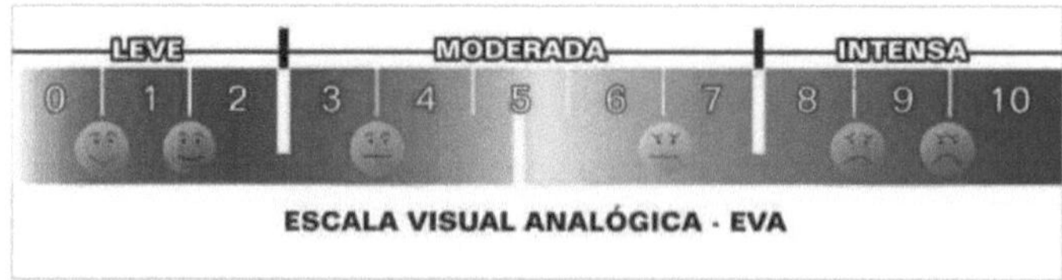

Figure 7: Pain intensity scale (0 to 10 points)

The clinical state of wound healing was also checked in terms of pain, heat, redness and oedema. Secretions from the surgical site were collected using a swab in culture medium (Figure 8), and the procedures of applying 0.1% methylene blue for five minutes on the experimental side, applying the laser for 60 seconds, irrigating with saline solution, collecting material using a swab again and irrigating again were repeated. On the control side, the material was collected with a swab in culture medium, the application of 0.1% methylene blue for five minutes was simulated, the laser was applied for 60 seconds, and all the other procedures were simulated.The swab, which has culture medium suitable for maintaining the same conditions for 24 hours, was immediately sent for laboratory examination.

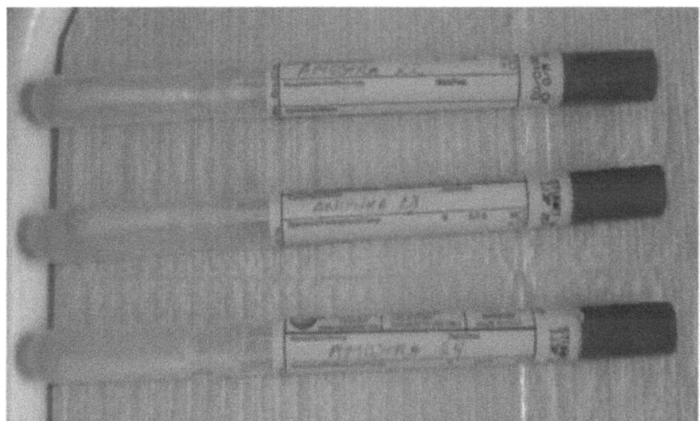

Figure 8: Swab samples with culture medium for transport

The patients were instructed to return in seven days to have the sutures removed (Figures 9 and 10).

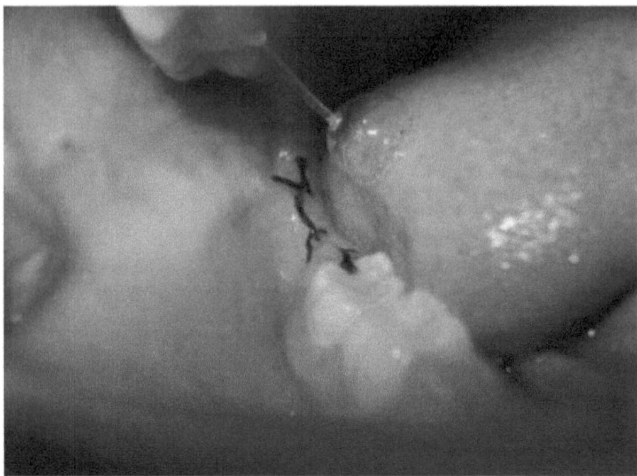
Figure 9: Experimental side, after one week

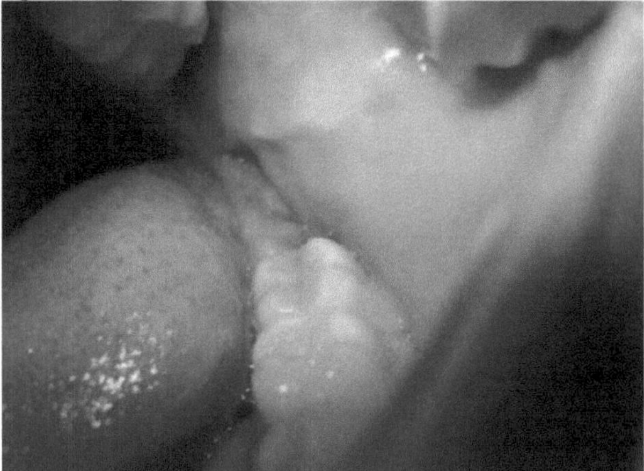
Figure 10: Control side, after one week, showing little oedema

All the secretion samples collected were immediately sent to a specialised laboratory for culture.

In the laboratory, the blood culture samples are placed in an appropriate oven at 36° C and shaken every 24 hours (Figures 11 and 12). The colour of the liquid in each of the flask is checked at the time of shaking and, if there is a different colour, it means that there has been bacterial growth. A little of the liquid is then collected and spread over three different agar plates (Figure 13) to identify and count the microorganisms where there has been growth (Figure 14).

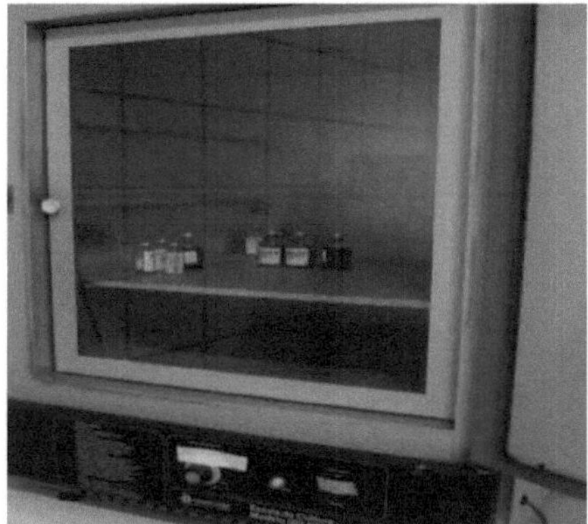

Figure 11: Oven with blood culture samples at 36° C

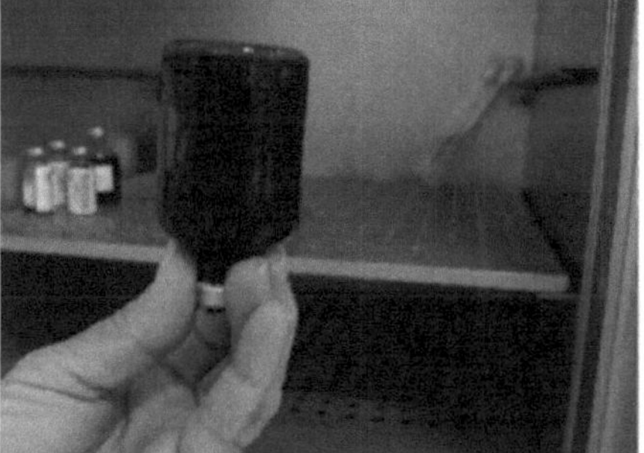

Figure 12: Samples (blood culture), shaken every 24 hours

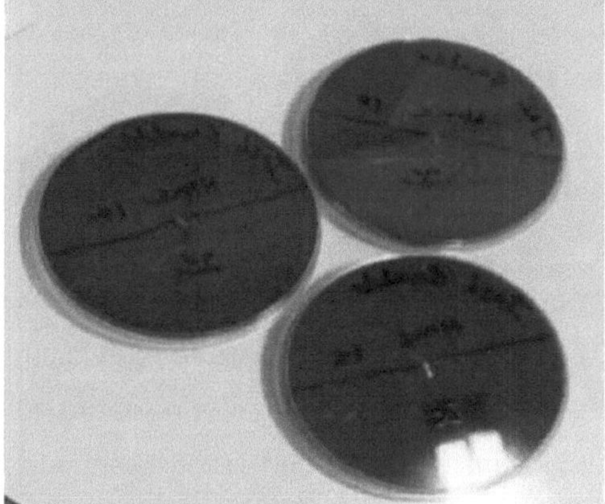

Figure 13: Samples in agar medium

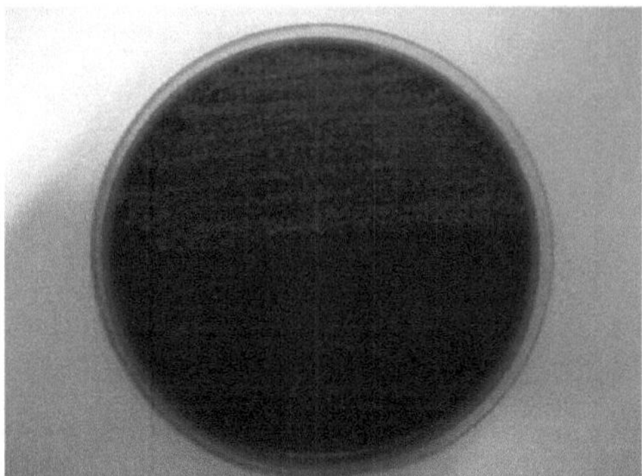

Figure 14: Sample where microorganisms grew

4.3 Evaluation method

Both sides, experimental and control, were analysed before surgery, in the immediate post-operative period, after 24 hours, and after seven days.

The study for comparison depended on the results found in the identification and counting of microorganisms by the laboratory
The results of the specialised tests, both in blood cultures taken immediately after extraction and in secretion cultures (after 24 hours). It also depended on patients' reports of pain and visual quality to determine the quality of the oedema in each patient and surgery.

Pain symptomatology was detected using a numerical, analogue and verbal scale, the Jensen et al. scale (1986), from zero to ten points.

Pre-operative and post-operative digital photos were taken of both treated sides.

A comparative study was carried out on the side that underwent exodontia accompanied by the application of a red AlGaInP (Indium-Gallium-Aluminium Phosphide) low-intensity laser (LLLT), with a wavelength of 660 nm, a power of 40 mW, a beam area of 0.04 cm^2 and an Energy Density of 60 J/cm^2 , for 60 seconds, and on the side where photodynamic therapy associated with a red AlGaInP (Indium-Gallium-Aluminium Phosphide) low-intensity laser (LLLT) was used, with a wavelength of 660 nm, a power of 40 mW, and an Energy Density of 60 J/cm^2 (transverse axis) for 60 seconds. These applications were made immediately post-operatively and after 24 hours on both surgical sides. The data obtained was compared using statistical methods determined after analysing the normality of the results presented.

4.4 Statistical analysis

Initially, all the variables were analysed descriptively. The quantitative variables were analysed by looking at the minimum and maximum values and calculating the means, standard deviations and quartiles (25th percentile, median and 75th percentile). Absolute and relative frequencies were calculated for the qualitative variables.

Friedman's non-parametric test (ROSNER, 1986) was used to compare the three blood cultures and secretions, as the assumption of data normality was rejected.

The Friedman non-parametric test (ROSNER, 1986) was used to compare the VAS, as the assumption of normality of the data was rejected.

The Wilcoxon non-parametric test (ROSNER, 1986) was used to compare the two percentages of elimination of microorganisms and the oedema score, as the assumption of normality of the data was rejected.

For the graphical presentation of the data, the Box-plot graph was used, which shows some summary measures of a set of data, such as: mean, median, minimum value, maximum value, as well as any extreme values called outliers, represented by an asterisk (*).

The study involved 13 patients. The significance level used for the tests was 5%.

CHAPTER 5

RESULTS

Thirteen patients aged between 16 and 29 years were assessed (mean 22.15 years, standard deviation 3.93 years and median 23 years). Eleven (84.6%) patients were female.

The patients were named patient 1, patient 2, patient 3, patient 4, patient 5, patient 6, patient 7, patient 8, patient 9, patient 10, patient 11, patient 12 and patient 13.

These patients underwent surgery on both the right and left sides of the mouth, with one side being called the experiment and the other the control. The surgeries on both sides were carried out at the same time, i.e. when the surgery on one side was finished, the surgery on the other side began immediately.

Blood samples were taken from the dental alveolus immediately after tooth extraction on the experimental and control sides and also after PDT (only on the experimental side).

The data obtained was analysed in two ways:

1- The first is the laboratory finding, with the quantification and classification of the microorganisms found.

2- The second was an analysis of the medical records to assess pain, which was properly assimilated and understood by the patients, using a visual analogue scale, which determines the pain the patient feels, on a horizontal line numbered from zero to ten, indicating the measure of their pain, from least intense to most intense. The medical records also recorded data on the presence of oedema, through visualisation.

In 11 patients (84.6%) the Klebs/ella sp microorganism was observed in the blood culture and in 2 patients *Escherichia coli* (15.4%).

The table below shows the results of the blood cultures taken immediately after extraction. Blood culture 1 was obtained on the experimental side and carried out in the first act, blood culture 2 on the control side, carried out in the second act, and blood culture 3 immediately after tfd (experimental side), carried out in the first act.

Patient	Microorganism	Blood culture	Blood culture 2	Blood culture 3
1	*Klebsiella sp*	400.000	300.000	100.000
2	*Klebsiella sp*	500.000	400.000	300.000
3	*Klebsiella sp*	500.000	400.000	300.000
4	*Klebsiella sp*	500.000	400.000	300.000
5	*Escherichia coli*	300.000	200.000	150.000
6	*Escherichia coli*	400.000	200.000	Rare
7	*Klebsiella sp*	500.000	350.000	150.000
8	*Klebsiella sp*	Countless	300.000	No growth
9	*Klebsiella sp*	450.000	Insufficient	200.000
10	*Klebsiella sp*	500.000	300.000	100.000
11	*Klebsiella sp*	500.000	240.000	100.000
12	*Klebsiella sp*	450.000	380.000	200.000
13	*Klebsiella sp*	500.000	380.000	Rare

Table 1: Identification and count of microorganisms found in alveoli of lower third molars (tooth 48), immediately after exodontia (cfu/mL)

We can see that there are fewer microorganisms on the control side than on the experimental side. The experiment side was submitted to PDT before the control side. The table below shows the descriptive values of the three blood cultures.

Table 1: Mean values, standard deviation, minimum, maximum and quartiles (25th percentile, median and 75th percentile) of the values obtained in the blood cultures carried out

Blood culture	Average	dp	Minimum	Maximum	P25	Median	P75
1	500000,00	162018,52	300000,00	Incont*	425000,00	500000,00	500000,00
2	320833,33	76093,05	200000,00	400000,00	255000,00	325000,00	395000,00
3	146154,00	110795,27	S. cresc.	300000,00	50000,50	150000,00	250000,00

Caption:

Dp: standard deviation Incont: uncountable

S.Cres: no growth

The Friedman non-parametric test showed that there was a significant difference between the blood cultures ($p < 0.001$). We observed a significant decrease from blood culture 1 to 3 ($p < 0.05$) and from blood culture 2 to 3 ($p < 0.05$). We also observed a significant difference between blood cultures 1 and 2 ($p < 0.05$), with blood culture 2 showing significantly lower values than blood culture 1.

The following graph shows the box-plot of this data.

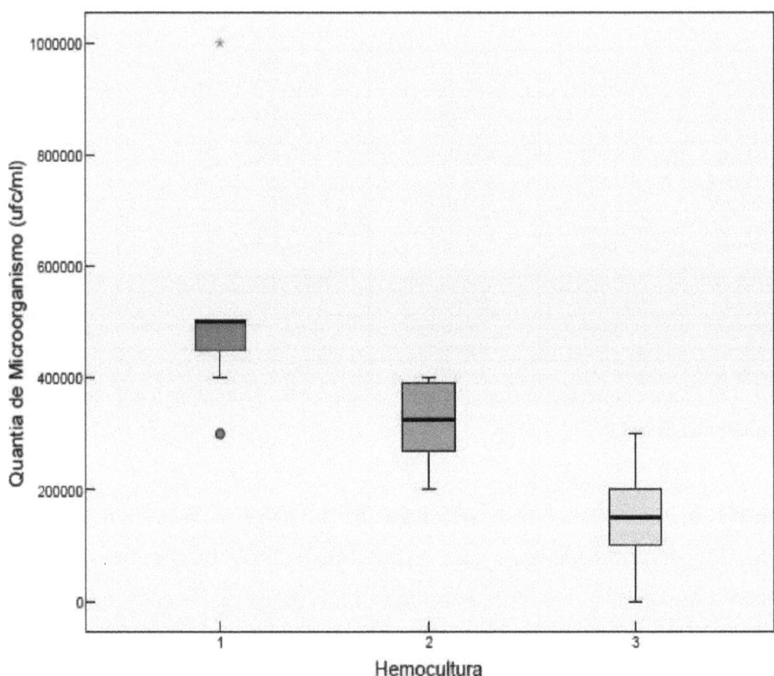

Graph 1: Box-plot of the amount of microorganisms found in lower third molar alveoli (tooth 48), immediately after extraction

The table below shows the percentages of elimination of microorganisms from blood cultures 1 and 3 (pre- and post-PDT) and blood cultures 2 and 3 (control and post-PDT).

Patient	Microorganism	% elimination of Hemoultura 1 and 3	% elimination of blood culture 2 and 3
1	*Klebsiella sp*	75,0	66,7
2	*Klebsiella sp*	40,0	25,0
3	*Klebsiella sp*	40,0	25,0
4	*Klebsiella sp*	40,0	25,0
5	*Escherichia coli*	50,0	25,0
6	*Escherichia coli*	Almost all	Almost all
7	*Klebsiella sp*	70,0	57,1
8	*Klebsiella sp*	100,0	100,0
9	*Klebsiella sp*	55,6	Indefinable
10	*Klebsiella sp*	80,0	66,7
11	*Klebsiella sp*	80,0	58,3
12	*Klebsiella sp*	55,6	47,4
13	*Klebsiella sp*	Almost all	Almost all

Table 2: Percentage elimination of microorganisms found in lower third molar alveoli (tooth 48)

Table 2: Mean, standard deviation, minimum, maximum and quartile values (25th percentile, median

and 75th percentile) of the % elimination in the blood cultures carried out

% of disposal	Average	dp	Minimum	Maximum	P25	Median	P75
Haemoc. 1 e 3	68,02	22,86	40,00	100,00	45,00	70,00	89,50
Blood 2 and 3	57,85	29,77	25,00	100,00	25,00	57,74	90,93

Using the non-parametric Wilcoxon test, we found that the % elimination from blood culture 1 to 3 was significantly higher than from blood culture 2 to 3 (p=0.007). The graph below shows the box-plot of this data.

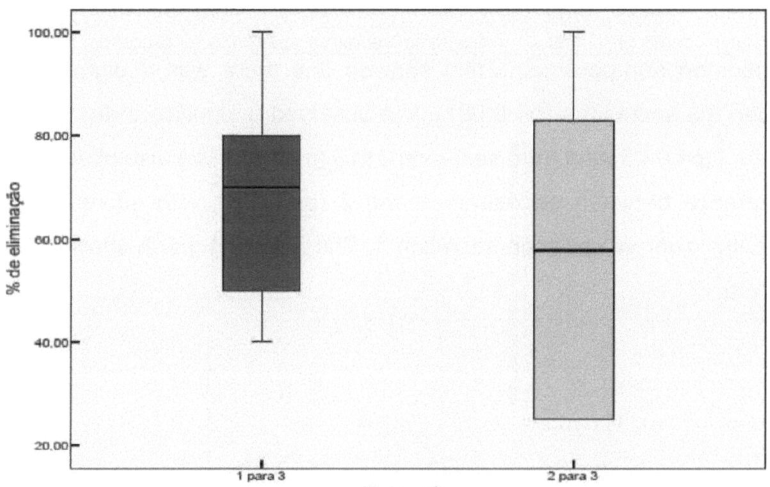

Graph 2: Box-plot of the % elimination of microorganisms found in lower third molar alveoli (tooth 48), immediately after exodontia

The following table shows the results of the secretions obtained the day after the extraction. Secretion 1 was obtained on the experimental side during the first procedure, secretion 2 on the control side during the second procedure and secretion 3 on the post-tfd (experimental side) during the first procedure.

Patient	Microorganism	Secretion 1	Secretion 2	Secretion 3
1	*Klebsiella sp*	500.000	380.000	100.000
2	*Klebsiella sp*	500.000	400.000	280.000
3	*Klebsiella sp*	Countless	500.000	300.000
4	*Klebsiella sp*	500.000	400.000	280.000
5	*Escherichia coli*	450.000	230.000	150.000
6	*Escherichia coli*	450.000	250.000	100.000
7	*Klebsiella sp*	500.000	400.000	200.000
8	*Klebsiella sp*	Countless	300.000	Rare
9	*Klebsiella sp*	500.000	400.000	250.000
10	*Klebsiella sp*	Countless	500.000	300.000
11	*Klebsiella sp*	500.000	300.000	100.000
12	*Klebsiella sp*	470.000	400.000	250.000
13	*Klebsiella sp*	500.000	380.000	100.000

Table 3: Identification and count of microorganisms found in alveoli of mandibular third molars (tooth 48), the day after extraction (cfu/mL)

We can see that we have lower quantities of microorganisms on the control side compared to the case side. The case side was submitted to PDT before the control side. The table below shows the descriptive values of the three blood cultures.

Table 3: Mean values, standard deviation, minimum, maximum and quartiles (25th percentile, median and 75th percentile) of the values obtained in the secretions

Secretion	Average	dp	Minimum	Maximum	P25	Median	P75
1	605384.62	225743,78	450000,00	Countless	485000,00	500000.00	750000,00
2	372307.69	82780,22	230000,00	500000,00	300000,00	400000.00	400000.00
3	185384.69	98962.41	Rare	300000.00	100000.00	200000.00	280000.00

The Friedman non-parametric test showed that there was a significant difference between the secretions (p< 0.001). We observed a significant decrease from secretion 1 to 3 (p< 0.05) and from secretion 2 to 3 (p< 0.05). We also observed a significant difference between secretions 1 and 2 (p< 0.05), with secretion 2 showing significantly lower values than secretion 1. The following graph shows the box-plot of this data.

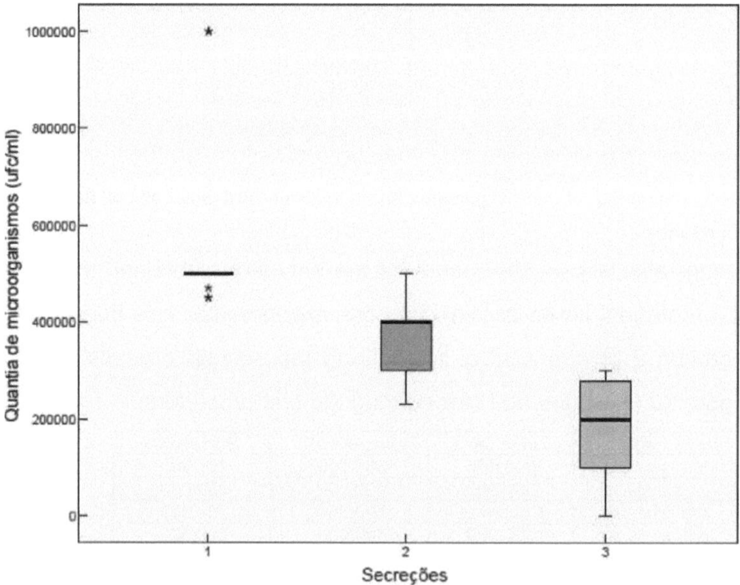

Graph 3: Box-plot of the amount of microorganisms found in the alveoli of lower third molars (tooth 48) the day after extraction

The following table shows the percentages of elimination of microorganisms from secretions 1 and 3 (pre and post PDT) and secretions 2 and 3 (control and post PDT).

Patient	Microorganism	% elimination of secretion 1 and 3	% elimination of secretion 2 and 3
1	*Klebsiella sp*	80,0	73,7
2	*Klebsiella sp*	44,0	30,0
3	*Klebsiella sp*	Indefinable	40,0
4	*Klebsiella sp*	44,0	30,0
5	*Escherichia coli*	66,7	34,8
6	*Escherichia coli*	77,8	60,0
7	*Klebsiella sp*	60,0	50,0
8	*Klebsiella sp*	Almost all	Almost all
9	*Klebsiella sp*	50,0	37,5
10	*Klebsiella sp*	Indefinable	40,0
11	*Klebsiella sp*	80,0	66,7
12	*Klebsiella sp*	46,8	37,5
13	*Klebsiella sp*	80,0	73,7

Table 4: Percentage elimination of microorganisms found in lower third molar alveoli (tooth 48)

Table 4: Mean, standard deviation, minimum, maximum and quartile values (25th percentile, median and 75th percentile) of the % elimination in the blood cultures carried out

% elimination	Average	dp	Minimum	Maximum	P25	Median	P75
Secretion 1 and 3	66,20	18,56	44,00	99,00	46,81	66,67	80,00
Secretion 2 and 3	51,76	21,22	30,00	99,00	36,14	40,00	70,18

Using the non-parametric Wilcoxon test, we observed that the % of elimination from secretion 1 to 3 was significantly higher than from secretion 2 to 3 (p=0.005). The graph below shows the box-plot of this data.

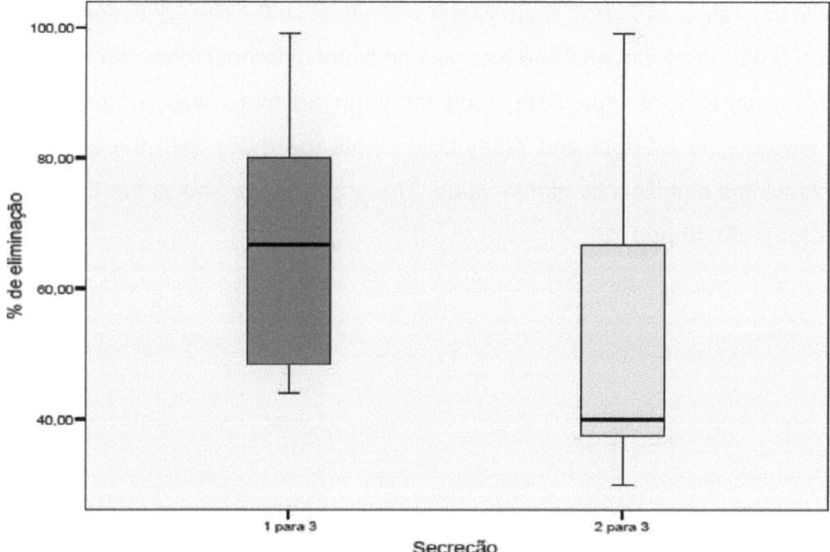

Graph 4: Box-plot of the % elimination of microorganisms found in lower third molar alveoli (tooth 48), the day after exodontia

Pain manifestations were measured 24 hours and 7 days after extraction in tooth 48 (treated with PDT) and tooth 38 (not treated with PDT) using the VAS. The values observed are shown in the table below:

Table 5: VAS values 24 hours and 7 days after extraction on teeth 48 and 38

Patient	Tooth 48		Tooth 38	
	24 hours	7 days	24 hours	7 days
1	0,0	0,0	3,0	0,0
2	0,0	0,0	1,0	0,0
3	1,0	0,0	2,0	0,0
4	0,0	0,0	2,0	0,0
5	0,0	0,0	1,2	0,0
6	0,0	0,0	1,0	0,0
7	0,5	0,0	1,5	0,0
8	0,0	0,0	2,5	0,0
9	0,5	0,0	2,5	0,0
10	0,0	0,0	2,0	0,0
11	0,0	0,0	2,0	0,0
12	0,0	0,0	3,0	0,0
13	0,0	0,0	3,0	0,0

The Friedman non-parametric test showed that there was a significant difference between the values presented above ($p < 0.001$). At 24 hours, the scores for tooth 48 differed significantly from those for tooth 38 ($p < 0.05$), showing a significantly lower value. At 7 days there was no significant difference between teeth 48 and 38 ($p > 0.05$). For tooth 48 there was no significant difference between the 24-hour and 7-day time points ($p > 0.05$), and for tooth 38 there was a significant difference between the 24-hour and 7-day time points ($p < 0.05$), with the 24-hour time point showing a significantly higher value. The graph below shows the 24-hour VAS scores for teeth 48 and 38.

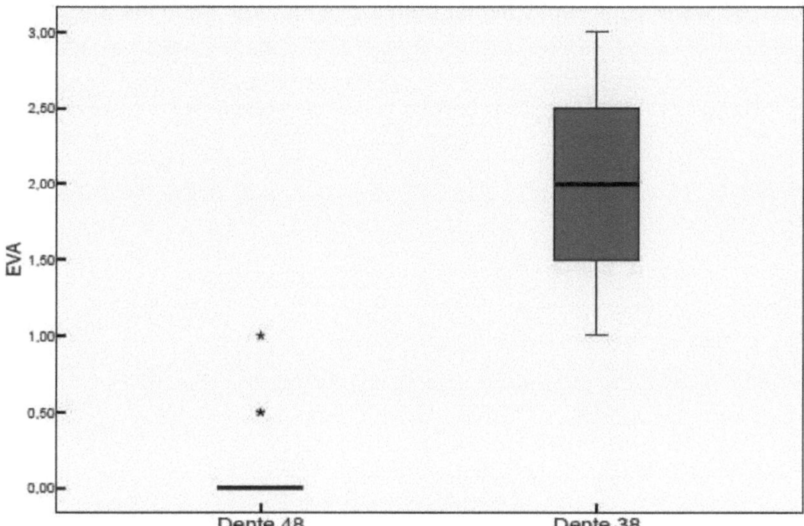

Graph 5: Box-plot of the 24-hour VAS on teeth 48 and 38

Oedema was observed 24 hours after extraction in teeth 48 and 38. For this classification, a scale of 0 to 5 was used, where:

0- absent

1- little, internal

2- barely visible, external

3-very visible, external

4-intense

5-very intense

Table 6: Score for the presence of oedema 24 hours after extraction in teeth 48 and 38

Patient	Tooth 48	Tooth 38
1	0	2
2	0	0
3	0	1
4	0	0
5	0	1
6	0	0
7	0	1
8	0	2
9	0	1
10	0	1
11	0	0
12	0	2
13	0	1

Using the non-parametric Wilcoxon test, we found a significant difference between the swelling scores of teeth 48 and 38 (p=0.006). We observed that the scores for tooth 38 were significantly higher than those for tooth 48 in the majority of patients.

CHAPTER 6

DISCUSSION

The results show a significant difference in the survival of microorganisms of the oral flora, given the situations to which the dental alveoli were subjected after exodontia. It points to a large reduction in immediate growth after the use of 0.1% methylene blue associated with the point application of low intensity laser light (LLLT) red, Twin Flex (MM Optics) AlGaInP (Indium-Gallium-Aluminium Phosphide), with a wavelength of 660 nm, power of 40 mW, beam area of 0.04 cm^2 and energy density of 60 J/cm^2 for 60 seconds.

It also shows that, between the time of extraction and the following day, the microorganisms found in secretions (24 hours) are the same as those found in blood cultures, and that there was growth in the oral flora between the act after PDT on the day of extraction and the act before PDT on the control day (24 hours). However, after PDT, in both situations, there was a drastic reduction in the number of colonies found.

Another fact that draws attention concerns the collection of material for blood culture. The post-PDT experimental side took place moments before the tooth on the control side (without PDT) was extracted, and the material collected for blood culture on the control side had fewer colonies than on the pre-PDT experimental side. The lower number of colonies on the control side could be explained by the fact that methylene blue may have come into contact with the oral cavity during the extensive irrigation of the alveolus of the tooth on the experimental side, which could even eliminate the microorganisms on the control side, given the uniformity of the data found. But this is just a hypothesis that could be further investigated in the future.

Phenothiazines have been widely studied as agents to mediate photoinactivation and also to mediate the elimination of neoplastic cells in mammals (HAMBLIN, 2004). In our study, methylene blue with subsequent laser irradiation, despite demonstrating a bactericidal effect on the bacteria found in the dental alveoli of the individuals reported in this study, was not effective against these microorganisms, as it reduced bacterial survival by approximately 50% when compared to the pre-TFD samples and the control side. The same can be said for the results found after 24 hours, despite the fact that there was growth of microorganisms in the oral flora of the patients in the study between the first 24 hours studied.

Tooth extraction wounds heal in a way that is no different from the healing of other wounds in the body, except for the particular anatomical location that exists after the tooth has been removed; the situation determined by the first 24 hours after the injury is important in the way healing occurs. For Manjo and Joris (1996), the presence of bacteria, the degree of blood supply, the nature of the wound (open or closed), the amount of dead tissue to be eliminated, the type of tissue injured and other factors determine how healing will occur. It should be noted that healing is best when the wound is closed, sutured and not infected, where the healing process progresses directly to the production of a scar.

By eliminating bacteria through the release of singlet oxygen produced by applying the laser to the 0.1% methylene blue dye, PDT helps to improve wound healing, as there was a reduction in bacteria at the site in the first few hours after surgery. This can also be seen from the analysis of the pain and oedema presented by the patients in our study, on the side treated with PDT, compared to the side where methylene blue was not applied.

Several authors have reported that oral pathologies such as caries, pulpitis, periodontal disease and ulcerated oral mucosa infections are accessible and susceptible to PDT. Komerick and Macrobert (2006) point out that there is a balanced native microflora in the oral cavity, and that PDT could potentially be a problem because it could lead to the growth of opportunistic microorganisms by selectively eliminating certain pathogens. However, in our study, the collection of material from the dental alveolus shortly after the lower third molars were extracted, prior to treatment with PDT (Blood Culture 1), proves that there was already a predominance of certain bacteria in that location.

As for the microorganisms, it is noteworthy that those found in the dental alveoli of extracted teeth are not those commonly involved in caries, such as *Streptococcus* or *Enterococcus* (TANZER, 1995) and/or periodontitis, such as *Actinobacillus, Porphyromonas, Prevotela, Bacteroides, Fusobacterium,*

Treponema, Enterococcus, Actinomes, (SLOTS, RAMS 1998) among others common in oral flora. But only *Klebsiella sp Esc,h2%)* and *Escherichia Coli* (15,38%).

The *Klebsiella* genus has biochemical characteristics that allow it to be identified: negative oxidase reaction, ferments glucose, reduces nitrate, positive lysine, negative citrate and indole, positive triple sugar iron (TSI) with gas production, negative ornithine, metabolises lactose, uses citrate as a carbon source and also hydrolyses urea, forming gas or not. Most samples are capable of producing butylene glycol as the end product of glucose fermentation (PODSCHUN et aL, 1992; GALES, 1997; KONEMAN et al., 2001). Although microorganisms of the *Klebsiella* genus are found in almost all natural environments and were not initially associated with infections, clinical isolates related to infections causing sepsis have been described (ROLLINS and JOSEPH, 2000).

Both *Klebsiella sp* and *Escherichia Coli* were found in the microbiota isolated from oral mucosa and carious cavities by Okoje et al. (2006). Souto et al. (2006), analysing the prevalence of "non-oral" pathogenic bacteria in the subgingival dental biofilm of patients with chronic periodontitis, found *Enterococcus faecalis* and *Escherichia coli,* among others, more frequently and at higher levels than in patients in the periodontally healthy group.

Similarly, Pimenta et al. (2006), when analysing the oral flora of children, found 16% of *Klebsiella pneumoniae and* 2.3% of *Escherichia Coli,* as well as S. *aureus (5%) and Coagulase Negative Staphylococci* (30%), drawing attention to the presence of *Staphylococcus sp* and *Klebsiella pneumoniae* in the mouth, as they can act as supplementary microbiota and cause oral or systemic disease.

In ICU patients, Oliveira et al. (2007) found 13.3% of *Kleibsella pneumoniae* and 3.3% of *Escherichia coli (E.coli)* when investigating the presence of respiratory pathogens in the oral cavity. In these patients, 70% of these bacteria were found in dental biofilm, 63.33% in tongue samples, 73.33% in artificial respirator tube samples and 43.33% in all areas simultaneously.

Bacteria present in dental biofilm that can colonise the oropharyngeal cavity (WIKSTROM, LINDE, 1986; GIBBONS, 1989; JOHANSON et al., 1969) have been studied since the 1970s, and three possible mechanisms have been described for associating oral biofilm with respiratory infections:

1) high concentration of pathogens in saliva may be due to poor oral hygiene (SOCRANSKY et al, 1963; CONTRERAS, SLOTS, 2000) and these pathogens could be aspirated into the lungs in large quantities, deteriorating immune defences (MANGANIELLO et al, 1977; SCANNAPIECO et al, 1992);

2) the oral biofilm could harbour colonies of lung pathogens and promote their growth (FUXENCH-LOPEZ, RAMIREZ- RONDA, 1978; WIKSTROM, LINDE, 1986) under specific conditions;

3) there would be greater ease of comolisation of the upper airways by pulmonary pathogens due to the presence of bacteria
present in oral biofilm (MOJON, 2002; SCANNAPIECO et al., 2003).

The determining factor for bacterial colonisation is the adhesion of bacteria to surfaces, with *Pseudomonas aeruginosa* and *Klebsiella pneumoniae* adhering more easily to the epithelial cells of hospitalised patients than non-hospitalised patients (JOHANSON et al, 1979; JOHANSON et al, 1980).

The presence of respiratory pathogens in the oral biofilm of ICU patients can serve as a reservoir for microorganisms associated with nosocomial pneumonia, according to Fourrier et al (1998) and Oliveira et al (2007).

For other authors (WIKSTROM, LINDE, 1986; FRANDSEN et al., 1987; FOURRIER et al., 1998; MARIK, CAREAU, 1999), inadequate oral hygiene concomitant with the use of drugs can alter salivation capacity and pH, facilitating an increase in the amount of bacteria in the oral biofilm of hospitalised patients during their metabolism.

Among all hospital-acquired infections, nosocomial pneumonia accounts for 10% to 15% of this total; and 20% to 50% of all patients affected by infections die (OLIVEIRA et aL, 2007). K. *pneumoniae* is responsible for a high mortality rate, according to Santos (2007).

K. pneumoniae has been isolated from the mouth of individuals with or without periodontal disease and in the oropharynx of asymptomatic carriers, where it is a source of lung infections in patients debilitated by alcoholism, diabetes and chronic lung diseases (SANTOS, 2007).

Among the pathogens related to hospital infections, *Klebsiella sp* has a high prevalence and can cause infections in any area of the body. This bacterium is the most frequently isolated aetiological agent in respiratory infections, especially in ICU patients, where it is responsible for 14% of primary bacteraemias, 10% of all bloodstream infections, 29% of experimental sepsis, 45% of wound infections, 6-8% of community-acquired pneumonia and 28% of all pneumonia (PITTET et aL, 1995; MARRA, 2002; PATERSON etaL, 2003).

Infections caused by *Klebsiella sp* are worrying because these microorganisms can acquire resistance to multiple drugs (HANSON et al., 1999; GUZMÁN-BLANCO et al., 2000; BUSH, 2001; THOMSON, 2001; BABIC, 2006), as well as being an important source of transmission of resistance between microorganisms of unrelated species, and represents an important source of bacterial dissemination in the hospital environment (JONES, 2000; PATERSON, 2006); which facilitates the risk of recurrence of outbreaks and/or the expression of other mechanisms of resistance to other classes of antimicrobials (BUISSON et al., 1987; ASENSIO et al., 2000; GNIADKOWSKI, 2001).

This resistance to antimicrobials continues to be the main growing cause of morbidity, mortality, length of stay and the need to use more toxic and expensive antimicrobials, resulting in increased hospital costs (JARVIS, 1996; SHLAES et al., 1997; MURTHY, 2001; PATTERSON, 2001).

In ICUs, these risk factors are well known and are related to the severity of the clinical conditions of patients, who are generally subjected to various invasive procedures, favouring access by microorganisms to the vascular system (PITTET et al., 1995; PENA et al., 1998; RICHARDS etaL, 1999).

Thus, 0.1% methylene blue associated with laser light, under the conditions described in this study, is effective in eliminating bacteria such as *Klebsiella sp and Escherichia Coli,* as shown by the analysis carried out. In this way, it can contribute to reducing the rates of morbidity, mortality, length of stay and the need to use more toxic and expensive antimicrobials related to these bacteria in hospitalised patients. A protocol for the use of 0.1% methylene blue in PDT in the oral cavity of hospitalised patients could be the subject of further research, as it is effective in reducing these bacteria.

However, further research is needed so that this therapy can be indicated as an adjunct to the classic methods already used in hospitalised patients with diseases related to these bacteria, in order to avoid increasing resistance to the antimicrobials used.

As for the post-operative period, the most common complications related to third molar extraction described in the literature are haemorrhage, flap dehiscence, alveolitis and paresthesia (CARDOSO, 2008). In all the cases analysed in our study, there were no post-operative complications, despite the fact that both lower third molars were removed on the same day.

As for pain, the side treated with PDT (experimental) showed a statistically significant reduction in pain from the first day onwards, greater than the control side.

With regard to oedema, there were differences between the treated side and the control side, with the treated side showing no oedema at any time. The treated side also had a better scar appearance after seven days.

CHAPTER 7

CONCLUSIONS

The results allow for the following conclusions:

1- PDT with 0.1% methylene blue associated with LLLT proved to be effective and useful.

2- There was a reduction in the growth of bacterial colonies in the dental alveolus with the use of PDT, under the conditions described in this study.

3- There was a reduction in pain, oedema and trismus in the post-operative period of lower third molar extraction treated with PDT, and healing was facilitated.

4- PDT with 0.1% methylene blue effectively reduced the growth of *Klebsiella sp* AND *Escherichia Coli* colonies.

REFERENCES

Ackroyd R, Kelty C, Brown N, Reed M. The history of photodetection and photodynamic therapy. **Photochem Photobiol.** 2001 ;74:656-69.

Almeida JM, Garcia VG, Theodoro LH. Photodynamic therapy: an option in periodontal therapy. **Arquivos em Odontol.** 2006 Jul-Set;42(3):161-256.

Asencio A, Oliver A, Gonzáles DP, Baquero F, Pérez-Díaz JC, Ros P. Outbreak of a multidrug-resistant Klebsiella pneumoniae strain in an intensive care unit: antibiotic use as risk factor for colonisation and infection. **Clin Infect Dis.** 2000;30:55-60.

Athiré MM. **Reduction of the inflammatory process with the application of gallium aluminium arsenide laser (λ = 830nm) in the postoperative period of extraction of included or semi-included mandibular third molars** [dissertation].

São Paulo: Nuclear and Energy Research Institute, University of São Paulo; 2002.

Babic M, Hujer AM, Bomono RA. What's new in antibiotic resistance? focus on [3-lactamases. **Drug Resist Updates.** 2006;10:1016-32.

Baxter GD. **Therapeutic lasers:** theory and practice. Singapore: Churchill Livingstone. 1994.

Besselink GAJ, Van Engelenburg FAC, Ebbing IG, Hilarius PM, De Korte D, Verhoeven AJ. **Vox Sanguinis.** 2003;85:25.

Bortoluzzi MC, Manfro R, Poggere V, Silva RD. Incidence of fibrinolytic alveolitis, acute infection, oedema, and pain longer than two days after dental extraction. **Rev. Odonto Ciênc.** 2008;23(2):111-4.

Boyle RK, Dolphin D. Structure and biodistribution relationships of photodynamic sensitizers. **Photochem Photobiol.** 1996;64:469-85.

Brugnera Jr A, Pinheiro ALB. **Lasers in modern dentistry.** São Paulo: Pancast; 1988.

Bush K. New p-lactamases in gram-negative bacteria: diversity and impact on the selection of antimicrobial therapy. **Clin Infect Dis.** 2001;32:1085-9.

Bueno-Cavanillas A, Delgado-Rodriguez M, López-Luque A, Schaffino-Cano S, Gálvez-Vargas R. Influence of nosocomial infection on mortality rate in an intensive care unit. **Crit Care Med.** 1994;22:55-60.

Buisson CB, Philippon A, Ansquer M, Legrand P, Montraveis F, Durval J.Transferable enzymatic resistance to third generation cephalosporin during nosocomial outbreak of multidrug-resistant Klebsiella pneumoniae. The

Lancet.1987;342:193-8.

Calderhead RG. The Nd:YAG and GaAlAs lasers: a laser comparative analysis in pain therapy. In: ATSUMI K, NIMSAKUL N. **Laser.** Tokyo: Japan Society for Laser Medicine; 1981.

Calderoni AMP, Fajardo VP, Carvalho PSP. Incidence of suppurative alveolitis in the surgical treatment of third molars. J **Bras Clin Odontol Integr.** 2003;7(42):453-6.

Caliceti P. **Trattato di patologia e clinica otorinolaringologica.** Bologna: L. Capelli; 1948.

Camino Júnior R, Luz JGC. Alveolitis: prevention and treatment principles. **JBC J Bras Clin Odontol Integr.** 2003 May-Jun .

Cardoso CL, Ribeiro ED, Bernini GF, Freitas DS, Ferreira Jr O, SanfAna E. Late abscess after extraction of lower third molars: report of two cases. **Rev Cir Traumatol Buco-Maxilo-fac.** 2008 Jul-Sep;8(3): 17-24.

Carmo Filho JR. **Epidemiological, microbiological and clinical correlation of hospital-acquired infections in intensive care units caused by klebsiella pneumoniae** [thesis]. São Paulo: Federal University of São Paulo, Paulista School of Medicine; 2003.

Chiapasco M, De Cicco L, Marrone G. Side effects and complications associated with third molar surgery. **Oral Surg Oral Med Oral Pathol.** 1993;76:412-20.

Christensen PJ, Kutty K, Adiam RT, Taft TA, Kampschroer BH. Septic pulmonary embolism due to periodontal disease. **Chest.** 1993;104:1927-9.

Christoffersen K, Richtner NG. Clinicai, bacteriologic and patho-anatomic considerations in chronic tonsillitis. **Acta Oto-Laryng.** 1951;39:102-20.

Contreras A, Slots J. Herpesviruses in human periodontal disease. **J Periodontal Res.** 2000;35:3-16.

De Boer MP, Raghoebar GM, Stegenga B, Schoen PJ, Boering G. Complications after mandibular third molar extraction. **Quintes Internat.** 1995;26(11):779-84.

Demidova TN, Hamblin MR. Photodynamic therapy targeted to pathogens. **Int J Immunopathol Pharmacol.** 2004; 17(3):245-54.

Demidova TN, Hamblin MR. Effect of cell-photosensitizer binding and cell density on microbial photoinactivation. **Antimicrob Agents Chemother.** 2005;49(6):2329-35 .

Donato AC, Boraks S. **Clinical laser:** practical applications in odonto-stomatology. São Paulo: Robe; 1993.

Ferreira J. **Analysis of necrosis in photosensitised normal tissues after photodynamic therapy: an** in vivo study [dissertation]. Ribeirão Preto: Ribeirão Preto Medical School, SP; 2003.

Finegold SM. Aspiration pneumonia. **Rev Infect Dis.** 1991;13:(Suppl9):S737- S742.

Floyd RA, Schneider JE, Dittme DP. Methylene blue photoinactivation of RNA viruses. **Antiviral Research.** 2004;61:141-51.

Fontana CR. **Photodynamic therapy on periodontopathogenic bacteria in planktonic phase and in multi-species biofilm** [thesis]. Araraquara: Araraquara School of Dentistry, Universidade Estadual Paulista-UNESP; 2007.

Foshi F, Fontana CR, Ruggiero K, Riahi R, Vera A, Doukas AG, et al. Photodynamic inactivation of enterococcus faecalis in dental root canals in vitro. **Lasers Surg Med.** 2007 Dec;39(10):782-7.

Fourrier F, Duvivier B, Boutigny H, Russel-Delvallez M, Chopin C. Colonisation of dental plaque: a source of nosocomial infections in intensive care units patients. **Crit Care Med.** 1998;26 301-8.

Frandsen EV, Reinholdt J, Kilian M. Enzymatic and antigenic characterisation of immunoglobulin Ai proteases from bacteroides and capnocytophaga spp. **Infect Immun.** 1987;55:631-8.

Fukuda H, Batlle A, Riley P. Kinetics of porphyrin accumulation in cultured epithelial cells exposed to ALA. **Int J Biochem.** 1993;25:1407-1410.

Fuxench-Lopez Z, Ramirez-Ronda CH. Pharyngeal flora in ambulatory alcoholic patients: prevalence of gram-negative bacilli. **Arch Intern Med.** 1978;138:1815-6.

Gabrielli D, Belisle E, Severino D, Kowaltowski AJ, Baptista MS. Binding, aggregation and photochemical properties of methylene blue in mitochondrial suspensions. **Photochemistry and Photobiology.** 2004;79(3):227-32.

Gales AC, Bolmstrom A, Sampaio J, Jones RN, Sader HS. Antimicrobial susceptibility of klebsiella pneumoniae producing ESBL isolated in hospitals in BraziL Braz **J Infect Dis.** 1997;1:196-203.

Gales AC. **Prevalence, sensitivity to antimicrobials and molecular typing of extended-spectrum beta-lactamase-producing klebsiella pneumoniae samples** [dissertation]. São Paulo: Federal University of São Paulo, Paulista School of Medicine; 1997.

Gallagher J, Marley J. Infratemporal and submasseteric infection following extraction of a non-infected maxillary third molar. **Br Dent J.** 2003;194:307-9.

Garcez AS, Ribeiro MS, Nunez SC, Souza FR. Photodynamic therapy in dentistry: low-power laser for microbial reduction. **Rev APCD.** 2003 May-Jun;57(3):223-5.

Genovese W J. **Low intensity laser:** therapeutic applications in dentistry. São Paulo: Livraria e editora Santos; 2007.

Gibbons RJ. Bacterial adhesion to oral tissues: a model for infectious diseases. **J Dent Res.** 1989;68:750-60.

Girardi C, Grando LJ, Philippi CK, Calvo MCM. Radiographic and histopathological study of the pericoronal tissues of unerupted and partially erupted third molars. **Rev Odonto Ciência,** Fac. Odonto/PUCRS. 2004 Oct-Dec;19(46):301-9.

Gniadkowski M. Evolution and epidemiology of extended spectrum p- lactamases producing microorganisms. **Clin Microbiol Infect Dis.** 2001;7:597-608.

Goldman L. **The biomedical laser:** technology & clinical applications. New York: Springer Verlag; 1981.

Graziani **M. Oral and maxillofacial surgery.** Rio de Janeiro: Guanabara Koogan; 1976. Gregori C. **Cirurgia buco-dento-alveolar.** São Paulo: Sarvier; 2004.

Guzmán-Blanco M, Casellas JM, Sader HS. Bacterial resistance to antimicrobial agents in latin america: the giant is awakening. Emerg **Re- emerg Dis in Latin America.** 2000;14(1):67-81.

Haas R, Dortbudak O, Mensdorff-Pouilly N, Mailatah G. Elimination of bacteria on different implant surfaces through photosensitisation and soft laser: an in vitro study.

Clin Oral Impl Res. 1997;8(4):249-54.

Hamblin MR, Hassan T. Photodynamic therapy: a new antimicrobial approach to infectious desease? **Photochen Photobiol Sei.** 2004;3:436-50.

Hanson ND, Thomson KS, Moland ES, Sanders CC, Berthod G, Penn RG. Molecular characterisation of a multiply resistant klebsiella pneumoniae encoding extended spectrum β-lactamases and a plasmid-mediated AmpC. J **Antimicrob Chemother.** 1999;44(3):377-80.

Hashimoto MCE. **Bacterial reduction with blue light-emitting diode associated with the photosensitiser rhodamine acid B:** in vitro study on streptococcus mutans [dissertation]. São Paulo: IPEN, University of São Paulo; 2005.

Holland CS, Hindle MO. The influence of closure or dressing of third molar sockets on postoperativeswelling and pain. **Br J Oral Maxillofac Surg.** 1984;22:65-71.

Huang Q, Fu WL, Chen B, Huang JF, Zhang X, Xue Q. Inactivation of dengue virus by methylene blue/narrow bandwidth light system. **Journal of Photochemistry and Photobiology B: Biology.** 2004;77:39-43.

Huxley EJ, Viroslav J, Gray WR, Pierce AK. Pharyngeal aspiration in normal adults and patients with depressed consciousness. **Am J Med.** 1978;64:564- 8.

Ingham E. **Enterobacteriaceae;** 2000. [cited 2005 Oct 10]. Available from: http//: medic. med. uth .tmc.edu.

Itri R, coordinators. **Photodynamic Therapy:** photoactive molecule complexes and their applications. São Pedro, SP; 2002.

Jarvis WR. Selected aspects of the socioeconomic impact of nosocomial infections:

morbidity, mortality, cost and prevention. **Infect Control Hosp Epidem.** 1996; 17:552- 7.

Jensen M P, Karoly P, Braver S. The measurement of clinical pain intensity, a comparison of six methods. **Pain.** 1986 Oct;27(1):117-26.

Johanson WG, Pierce AK, Sanford JP. Changing pharyngeal bacterial flora of hospitalised patients. Emergence of gram-negative bacilli. **N Engl J Med.** 1969;281:1137-40.

Johanson Jr WG, Woods DE, Chaudhuri T. Association of respiratory tract colonisation with adherence of gram-negative bacilli to epithelial cells. J **Infect Dis.** 1979;139:667-73.

Johanson Jr WG, Higuchi JH, Chaudhuri TR, Woods DE. Bacterial adherence to epithelial cells in bacillary colonisation of the respiratory tract. **Am Rev Respir Dis.** 1980;121:55-63.

Jones KC, Silver J, Millar WS, Mandei L. Chronic submasseteric abscess: anatomic, radiologic, and pathologic features. AJNR. 2003;24:1159-63.

Jones R. Global incidence, types and screening of extended-spectrum p-lactamases. In: **1° Symposium ESBL:** incidence, importance and solutions.

Argentina; 2000.

Kirszberg C, Rumjanek VM, Capella MAM. Methylene blue is more toxic to erythroleukemic cells than to normal peripheral blood mononuclear cells: a possible use in chemotherapy. **Cancer Chemother, Pharmacol.** 2005;dec;56,(6):659-65.

Kohler B, Petterson BM, Bratthall D. Streptococcus mutans in plaque and saliva and the development of caries. **Scand J Dent Res.** 1981 Feb;89(1):19- 25.

Komerick N, Macrobert, AJ. Photodynamic therapy as an alternative antimicrobial modality for oral infections. **J Environ Pathol Toxicol Oncol.** 2006;25(1-2):487-504.

Koneman EW, Allen SD, Dowel Jr VR, Sommer HM. **Microbiological diagnosis:** text and colour atlas Enterobacteriaceae. 5th ed. Rio de Janeiro: MDSI; 2001. p. 177- 250.

Lambrechts SAG, Aalders MCG, Marle JV. Mechanistic study of the photodynamic inactivation of candida albicans by a cationic porphyrin. **Antimicrob Agents Chemother.** 2005 May;5(49):2026-34.

Larsen PE. Alveolar osteitis after surgical removal of impacted mandibular third molars. **Oral Surg Oral Med Oral Pathol.** 1992;73:393-7.

Lima MA. **Repair of delayed cutaneous wounds, submitted to treatment with low intensity laser, associated or not with photosensitising drug - histological study in rats** [dissertation]. Marília:

University of Marília; 2004.

Ma J, Jiang L. Photogenerastion of singlet oxygen and free radicals by tetrabrominated hypocrellin B derivate. **Free Radie Res.** 2001;35:767-77.

Machado AEH. Photodynamic therapy: principies, potential of application and perspectives. **Quím Nova.** 2000;23(2):237-43.

Madson B, Ofek I, Clegg S, Abraham SN. Type 1 fimbrial shafts of escherichia coli and klebsiella pneumoniae influence sugar binding specificities of their fimbre H adhesions. **Infect Immun.** 1994;62:843-8.

Maduro R. **Pathologie de TAmygdale.** Paris: Masson; 1953.

Maiman TH. Stimulated optical radiation in ruby. **Nature.** 1960; 187:93.

Majno G, Joris I. **Cells, tissues and disease:** principies of general pathology. USA: Blackwell Science; 1996. p. 465-82.

Malik Z, Hanania J, Nitzan Y. Bactericidal effects of photoactivated porphyrins-an alternative approach to antimicrobial drugs. **J Photochem Photobiol B.** 1990;5(3-4):281-93.

Manganiello AD, Socransky SS, Smith C, Propas D, Oram V, Dogon IL. Attempts to increase viable count recovery of human supragingival dental plaque. **J Periodontal Res.** 1977;12:107-9.

Manyak MJ. Photodynamic therapy: present concepts and future applications. **Cancer J.** 1990;3:104-9.

Marra AR. **Analysis of risk factors related to the lethality of hospital bloodstream infections caused by klebsiella pneumoniae** [dissertation]. São Paulo: Federal University of São Paulo, Paulista School of Medicine; 2002.

Marcotte H, Lavoei MC. Oral microbial ecology and the holi of salivary immunoglobulin A. **Microbiol Mol Biol Rev.** 1998 Mar;62(1):71-109.

Marik PE, Careau P. The role of anaerobes in patients with ventilator- associated pneumonia and aspiration pneumonia: a prospective study. **Chest.** 1999;115:178-83.

Marinho SA. **Effect of photodynamic therapy (PDT) on cultures of candida sp and epithelial cells: an** in vitro study [thesis]. Porto Alegre: Pontifical Catholic

University of Rio Grande do Sul; 2006.

Martorelli SBF, Cavalcanti PHH, Albuquerque RS, Marinho BVS, Guerra EC, Martorelli FO. Complex odontoma in the mandible: report of a clinical case associated with an included third molar crossed by the lower tooth.
Medicenter.com - Odontologia, 18.03.2004. [cited 17 Apr 2006]. Available from: http://www.odontologia.com.br/artigos.asp7idM46.

Marzola C, Nary Filho H, Kawakami RY, Rodrigues CBF. Retained mandibular third molars: aetiology, irruption accidents, classification and surgical technique. **Rev Odonto Ciência.** Fac. Odonto/PUCRS, 1990/2;5(10):9-25.

Marzola C. **Exodontic Technique.** São Paulo: Pancast; 1994. p 267-97.

Menezes PFC, Bernal C, Imasato H, Bagnato VS, Perussi JR. Photodynamic

activity of different dyes. **Laser Physics.** 2007;17(4):468-71.

Meisel P, Kocher T. Photodynamic therapy for periodontal diseases: State of the art. **J Photochem Photobiol B.** 2005;79(2): 150-70.

Mester E. A laser sugar alkamazaea a gyogyaezatban. **Orv Hetilap.** 1966;1007:1012.

Mian J, Berg K. The photodegradation of porphyrins in cells can be used to estimate the lifetine onf singlet oxygen. **Photochem Photobiol.** 1991 ;53:549- 53.

Mion D. **Antibacterial therapy in chronic palatine tonsillitis in adults, based on the antibiogram** [thesis]. São Paulo: Faculty of Medicine, University of São Paulo; 1965.

Mojon P. Oral health and respiratory infection. **J Can Dent Assoe.** 2002;68:340-5.

Moro LM, Gayotto, MV, Camargo Filho GP. Indications for lower third molar surgery. **Rev Inst Ciência e Saúde.** 2001 Jul-Dec;19(2):121- 125.

Morris JF, Sewell DL.Necrotising pneumonia caused by mixed infection with actinobacillus actinomycetemcomitans and actinomyces israelii: case report and review. **Clin Infect Dis.** 1994;18:450-2.

Muller F. **Antimicrobial photodynamic therapy against gram-positive bacteria: a** comparative study of photosensitising agents [dissertation]. São José dos Campos: Univap, Vale do Paraíba University; 2006.

Murthy R. Implementation of strategies to control antimicrobial resistance. **Chest.** 2001; 119(2):405S-11S.

Nascimento PM, Pinheiro AL, Salgado MA, Ramalho LM. A preliminary report on the effect of laser therapy on the healing of cutaneous surgical wounds as a consequence of an inversely proportional relationship between wavelength and intensity: histological study in rats. **Photomed. Laser Surg.** 2004 Dec;22(6):513-8.

Newbrun E, Matsukubo T, Hoover CI, Graves RC, Brown AT, Disney JA, et al. Comparison of two screening tests for streptococcus mutans and evaluation of their suitability for mass screenings and private practice. **Community Dent Oral Epidemiol.** 1984 Oct;12(5):325-31.

Nogueira AS, Ponzoni D, Pasinato E, Ferrari LK, Farias RD. Main disorders caused by impacted teeth. **Rev da APCD.** 1997 May-Jun;51(3):247-9.

Okoje, VN, Alonge TO, Adeyemi AT, Akinmoladun VI. **Oral** microbial isolates seem at dental clinic. In: The preliminary programme for 5th Annual Scientific Congress of

IARD; 2006. Nigeria: UCH Ibadan; 2006.

Oliveira LCBS, Carneiro PPM, Fisher, RG, Tinoco EMB. Presence of respiratory pathogens in the oral biofilm of patients with nosocomial pneumonia. **Rev Bras Terap Intens.** 2007 Oct-Dec;19(4):428-33.

Orth K Rúck A, Stanescu A, Beger HG. Intraluminal treatment of inoperable oesophageal tumours by intralesional photodynamic therapy with methylene blue. **Lancet.** 1995(345):519-20.

Peloi LS. **Studies of the application of methylene blue dye in photodynamic therapy** [dissertation]. Maringá: State University of Maringá; 2007.

Paterson DL. Resistance in gram-negative bacteria: enterobacteriaceae. **Am J Infect Control.** 2006;34:S20-8.

Patterson JE. Is there an effect on antimicrobial resistance? **Chest.** 2001 ;119:426S-30S.

Peacock EE, Van Winkle W. **Wound repairs.** Philadelphia: W.B. Saunders; 1976.

Pena C, Pujl M, Ardanuy C, Ricard A, Paliares R, Linares J, et al. Epidemiology and successful control of a large outbreak due to klebsiella pneumoniae producing extended spectrum betalactamases. **Antimicrob Agent Chemother.** 1998;1:53-8.

Paterson DL, Ko WC, Gotteberg AV, Casellas JM, Mulazimoglu L, Klugman KP, et al. Outcome of cephalosporin treatment for serious infections due to apparently susceptible organisms producing extended-spectrum 0- lactamases: implications for the clinical microbiology laboratory. **Antimicrob Agent Chemother.** 2001;39:2206-12.

Peterson LJ, Ellis E, Tucker MR. **Contemporary oral and maxillofacial surgery.** 4th ed. Rio de Janeiro: Elsevier Editora; 2005. p.252-53, 379-81.

Perussi JR. Photodynamic inactivation of microorganisms. **Quim Nova.**

2007;30(4):988-94.

Pimenta FC, Santiago SB, Lima ABM, Oliveira ACA, Lamaro-Cardoso J. **Isolation, counting and identification of mutans streptococci, staphylococci and gram negative rods in the saliva of children assisted by a social programme in the municipality of Senador Canedo-GO.** In: 6º Pan American Congress and 10th Brazilian Congress of Hospital Infection and Epidemiology, 2006; Porto Alegre: ABEV; 2006.

Pinto JR, Tanaka EE, Martins LP, Stabile GAV, Borges HOL Pericoronaritis related to recurrent tonsillitis: review of the literature and report of a case. **Rev Odonto Ciênc,** Fac. Odonto/PUCRS. 2005 Jan-Mar;20 (47):88- 92.

Pittet D, Wenzel, RP. Nosocomial bloodstream infections: secular trends in rates, mortality and contribution to total deaths. **Arch Intern Med.** 1995;155:1177-84.

Podschun R, Penner P, Ullman U. Interaction of klebsiella capsule type 7 with human polymorphonuclear leucocytes. **Microb Path.** 1992;13:371-9.

Pollack SV. Wound healing: a review I: the biology of wound healing. J **DermatSurg Oncol.** 1979;5(5):389-93.

Prates RA. **Malachite green as a photosensitiser in photodynamic therapy: bactericidal action on actinobacillus actinomycetemcomitans:** an in-vitro study [dissertation]. São Paulo: Nuclear and Energy Research Institute, University of São Paulo; 2005.

Prime J. **Les accidents toxiques par 1'eosinate de sodium.** Paris: Jouve and Boyer; 1901.

Raab O. Uber die wirkung fluoreszierender stoffe auf Infusorien. **Z. Biol.** 1900;39:524-46.

Ribeiro MS, Groth EB, Yamada Júnior AM, Garcez AS, Suzuki LC, Prates RA , et al. Antimicrobial photodynamic therapy. In: **Virtual book:** 23rd CIOSP, São Paulo, 2005, 26 p. [cited 10 Nov 2005]. Available from: http://www.netodonto.com.br/ciosp/index.php.

Ribeiro MS, Zezel DM. **Low-intensity laser:** dentistry and the laser. São Paulo: Quintessence Editora Ltda; 2004.

Richards MJ, Edwards JR, Culver DH, Gaynes RP. Nosocomial infections in paediatric intensive care units in the United States. **Pediatrics.** 1999;103:1-7.

Roolins DM, Joseph SW. **Enterobacteriaceae,** 2000. [cited 2005 Oct 12]. Available from: http//:medic.med.utm.tmc.edu.

Rosa OPS. Salivary levels of streptococcus mutans and lactobacilli and susceptibility to dental caries. **CECADE News.** 1994,Jan/Apr;2(1): 15-26.

Rosner B. **Fundamentais of biostatistics.** 2nd ed. Boston: PWS Publishers; 1986.

Sahly H, Aucken H, Benedi VJ, Forestien C, Fussing V, Hansen DS, et al. Impairment of respiratory burst in polymorphonuclear leukocytes by ESBL strains of klebsiella pneumoniae. **Pubmed-Medline University Hosp Schleswig Hotstein,** 241105 Liei Germany; 2002.

Santos DF. **Microbiological characteristics of klebsiella pneumoniae isolated in**

the hospital environment from patients with nosocomial infection [dissertation]. Goiânia: Catholic University of Goiás; 2007.

Santos SSF, Jorge AOC. In vitro antimicrobial susceptibility of enterobacteriaceae and pseudomanadaceae isolated from oral cavity. **Postgraduate Rev Fac Odontol S José dos Campos.** 1999 Jan;2(1):40-4.

Scannapieco FA, Stewart EM, Mylotte JM. Colonisation of dental plaque by respiratory pathogens in medical intensive care patients. **Crit Care Med.** 1992;20:740-5.

Scannapieco FA, Mylotte JM. Relationships between periodontal disease and bacterial pneumonia. J **Periodontol.** 1996;67(suppl 10): 1114-22.

Scannapieco FA, Bush RB, Paju S. Associations between periodontal disease and risk for nosocomial bacterial pneumonia and chronic obstructive pulmonary disease: a systematic review. **Ann Periodontol.** 2003;8:54-69.

Schwingel AR. **Antimicrobial photodynamic therapy in the treatment of candidosis in HIV-positive patients** [dissertation]. São Paulo: IPEN, São Paulo School of Dentistry, University of São Paulo; 2007.

Sinclair DG, Evans TW. Nosocomial pneumonia in the intensive care unit. **Br J Hosp Med.** 1994;51:177-80.

Shlaes DM, Gerding DN, John JF, Craig WA, Bornstein DL, Duncan RA ,et al. Society for healthcare epidemiology of america and infectious disease society

of america joint committee on the prevention of antimicrobial resistance: guidelines for the prevention of antimicrobial resistance in hospitals. **Infect ContrEpid.** 1997;18:275-91.

Simplíci FI, Maionchi F, Hioka N. Photodynamic therapy: pharmacological aspects, applications and recent advances in drug development. **Quim Nova.** 2002;25(5):801-7.

Slots J, Rams TE, Listgarten MA. Yeats, enteric rods and pseudomonas in the subgingival flora of severe adult perodontitis. **Oral Microb and Immunol.** 1998;3:47-52.

Socransky SS, Gibbons RJ, Dale AC, Bortnick L, Rosenthal E, MacDonald JB. The microbiota of the gingival crevice area of man: total microscopic and viable counts and counts of specific organisms. **Arch Oral Biol.** 1963;8:275- 80.

Soukos NS, Chen PS, Morris JT, Ruggiero K, Abernethy AD, Som S, et al. Photodynamic therapy for endodontic disinfection. **J Endod.** 2006 Oct;32(10):978-84.

Souto R, Arnaldo FBA, Uzeda M, Colombo APV. Prevalence of "non-oral" pathogenic bacteria in subgingival biofilm of subjects with chronic periodontitis. **Braz J Microbiol.** 2006 Sep;37(3):208-15.

Sternberg ED, Dolphin D. Pyrrolic photosensitizers. **Curr Medic Chem.** 1996;3:293-324.

Sternberg ED, Dolphin D, Bruckner C. Porphyrin-based photosensitizers for use in photodynamic therapy. **Tetrahedron.** 1998;54:4151-202.

Stockhausen G, Felbier R. Local treatment of external lesion with aminoacids and antibiotics. **Medsche Mschr Ltuttg.** 1972;26:225.

Tanzer JM. Dental caries is a transmissible infections disease, the keys and fitzegeral revikutin. **J Dental Res.** 1995;74:1536-42.

Tardivo JP, Giglio AD, Oliveira CS, Gabrielli DS, Junqueira HC, Tada DB, et al. Methylene blue in photodynamic therapy: from basic mechanisms to clinical applications. **Photodiag and Photodyn Ther.** 2005;2:175-91.

The committee for The Japanese Respiratory Society guidelines in management of respiratory infections. **Respirology.** 2004;9:S30-S34.

Thomson KS. Controversies about extended spectrum 0-lactamases and Amp C. **Emerg Infect Dis.** 2001 ;7(2): 333-6.

Toews GB. Nosocomial pneumonia. **Am J Med Sei.** 1986; 291:355-67.

Tomé FM. **Synthesis and stetrophotometric analysis of naphthalocyanines for application in photodynamic therapy** [dissertation]. São José dos Campos: Univap, Universidade do Vale do Paraíba, SP; 2002.

Vasconcellos RJH, Oliveira DM, Moreira MD, Fulco MHM. Incidence of retained third molars in relation to Winter's classification. **Rev Cir Traumat Buco- Maxilo-Facial.** 2002 Jan-Jun;2(1):43-7.

Vitti RP, Sverzut AT, Moraes M. **Etiological factors of alveolitis: a** retrospective study at the Piracicaba School of Dentistry FOP/UNICAMP from 1995 to 2003. In: 13th Internal Scientific Initiation Congress

Unicamp, 2005; Piracicaba School of Dentistry - FOP/UNICAMP, 2005.

Von Tappeiner H, Jesionek A. Therapeutische versuchen mit floreesziderenden stoffen. muench, **Med Wochenschr.** 1903;47:2042-4.

Von Tappeiner H, Jodlbauer A. Uber wirkung der photodynamischen floreesziderenden: stoffen auf protozoan und enzyme. **Dtsch Arch Klin Med.** 1904;80:427-87.

Wainwright M. Photodynamic antimicrobial chemotherapy (PACT). J **Antimicrob Chemother.** 1998;42(1): 13-28.

Wainwright M, Grice NJ, Pye LEC. Phenothiazine photosensitizers: bis(arylamino)phenothiazines. **Dyes and Pigments.** 1999 Apr;42;(Pt 2.3,7)45-51.

Wainwright M. Methylene blue derivatives: suitable photoantimicrobials for blood product disinfection? **International Journal of Antimicrobial Agents.** 2000;16:381-94.

Wainwright M. Pathogen inactivation in blood products. **Curr Med Chem.** 2002;9(1):127-43.

Walsh L J. The current status of low light laser therapy in dentistry: hard tissue applications. **Aust Dent J.** 1997;42(5):(Pt 2)302-6.

Wilson M, Dobson J, Harvey W. Sensitisation of oral bacteria to killing by low-power laser radiation. **Curr Microbiol** 1992;25(2):77-81.

Wilson BD, Mang TS, Stool H, Jones C, Cooper M, Dougherty TJ. Photodynamic therapy for treatment of basal cell carcinoma. **Arch Dermatol** 1992;128:1597-601.

Wikstrom M, Linde A. Ability of oral bacteria to degrade fibronectin. **Infect Immun.** 1986;51:707-11.

Zambon JJ. Periodontal diseases: microbial factors. In: American Academy of Periodontology. **Ann. Periodontology.** 1996;879-925.

Zancanela DC, Machado AEH; Oliveira CA; Contijo Filho PP. **Photoinactivation of s. aureus promoted by methylene blue and zinc phthalocyanine.** In: 29th Annual Meeting Soc Bras Quím; 2006. Águas de Lindóia; 2006.

ANNEX 1

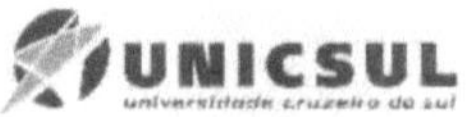

Comissão de Ética para Análise de Projetos de Pesquisa

<u>APROVAÇÃO</u>

A Comissão de Ética para Análise de Projetos de Pesquisa da Universidade Cruzeiro do Sul, <u>APROVOU</u> o protocolo n.º **122/2008**, intitulado: *"Estudo comparativo da ação da terapia fotodinâmica em exodontia."*, apresentado pela discente Sueli de Souza Costa, orientada pelo Prof. Walter João Genovese, do curso de Mestrado em Odontologia, bem com o Termo de Consentimento Livre e Esclarecido.

UNICSUL, 14 de Agosto de 2008.

Prof. Dr. Danilo Antonio Duarte
Presidente da Comissão de Ética

Observação: Cabe ao pesquisador elaborar e apresentar a Comissão de Ética, o relatório final sobre a pesquisa (RESOLUÇÃO DO CONSELHO NACIONAL DE SAÚDE Nº 196, 10/10/1996, inciso 9.2, letra "c")

ANNEX 2:
SIMPLIFIED MEDICAL RECORD

Name:<u>Birth</u>____// sex: F M

End. Res phone

Address Profession Phone

Identity No. ____

ANAMNESIS FORM/HEALTH QUESTIONNAIRE

Main complaint and evolution of the current illness

Do you suffer from any illnesses () yes () no. Which one(s)?

Are you currently undergoing medical treatment? ( ) yes ( ) no.

Pregnancy ( ) yes ( ) no

Are you using any medication () yes () no. Which ones?

Name of treating doctor/telephone number:_________________________________

Do you have any allergies () yes ( ) no. Which one(s)? _____________________________

Have you ever had an operation () yes () no. Which one(s)?_____________________

Did you have any problems with healing? ( ) yes ( ) no; with bleeding? ( ) yes ( ) no Did you have any

problems with anaesthesia? () yes () no

Do you suffer from any of the following illnesses?

Rheumatic fever ( ) yes ( ) no;   heart problems () yes () no

Kidney problems ( ) yes ( ) no;   stomach problems () yes () no

Respiratory problems () yes () no; allergic problems () yes () no diabetes () yes () noHypertension   ()

yes () no;

Joint problems or rheumatism () yes () no; habits _______________________________

Family history ____

Other important observations ____

I DECLARE THAT THE INFORMATION PROVIDED ABOVE IS COMPLETELY TRUE.

Place and datePatient   's or legal guardian's signature

ANNEX 3:

Authorisation to carry out the treatment

Me .... ID

.... CPF   below I sign, I give my full consent to

.... Drpararealise   PHOTODYNAMIC THERAPY

with a low-intensity AlGaInP (Indium-Gallium-Aluminium Phosphide) laser.

I freely and voluntarily authorise the treatment and therapy presented to me, of which I have received clear, simple explanations and have understood the purposes, as well as knowing that the treatments follow the appropriate technical and scientific principles recognised by dentistry. I declare that I have had the opportunity to ask questions about the importance of this procedure and about current research and treatment alternatives.

I authorise the taking of X-rays and photographs for scientific and didactic purposes, provided that my privacy is protected throughout the service and that my oral conditions are not unnecessarily exposed.

Place, date: .... from ....

Signature of patient or legal guardian ....

Identity document ....

NOTE: For patients considered to be minors, incapacitated or relatively civilly capable, the signature of a responsible person of legal age and duly documented, proving that they are legally responsible for the patient, is required.

ANNEX 4:

Laser therapy clinical records

Start date: _________________ // ______

Probable clinical diagnosis: ....

Procedures carried out: ....

1- Parameters:...

2-Session immediately after the microbiota culture (1° day)

3- Clinical follow-up 7° day:

Report:...

Clinical/laboratory results: ....

Date: ....

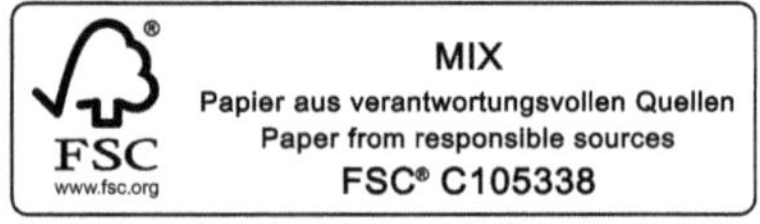